MANUAL OF NERVE CONDUCTION VELOCITY TECHNIQUES

Manual of Nerve Conduction Velocity Techniques

Joel A. DeLisa, M.D., M.S.

Associate Chief of Staff/Education
Assistant Chief for Rehabilitation Medicine Service
Seattle Veterans Administration Center
and
Associate Professor, Department of Rehabilitation Medicine
University of Washington
Seattle, Washington

Keith Mackenzie, M.D., M.S.

Associate Director
Sacred Heart Rehabilitation Center
Spokane, Washington

Raven Press ■ New York

Raven Press, 1140 Avenue of the Americas, New York, New York 10036

Made in the United States of America

Library of Congress Cataloging in Publication Data
Main entry under title:

Manual of nerve conduction velocity techniques.

Bibliography: p.
Includes index.
1. Neural conduction—Measurement. 2. Electrodiagnosis.
3. Electromyography. I. DeLisa, Joel A. II. Mackenzie, Keith. [DNLM: 1. Neural conduction. 2. Electrodiagnosis. WL 102.7 M294]
RC77.M28 616.8′707547 81-40021
ISBN 0-89004-656-5 AACR2

Second Printing, February 1983

Preface

This manual is designed to help physicians in electrodiagnosis training and electromyographers in practice to develop consistent techniques for performing motor and sensory nerve conduction velocity and latency studies, as well as repetitive stimulation of motor nerves. It also provides ready access to standardized values for these studies and serves as a reference when studying nerves not commonly tested. The manual is developed for use in the electrodiagnosis laboratory and is not intended to replace standard tests and literature references.

Descriptions of each nerve conduction technique follow the same sequence, beginning with the placement site for the active electrode, followed by sites for the reference electrode, the ground electrode, and the stimulating cathode and anode. Typical electromyograph equipment settings (frequency, sweep speed, and gain) are noted, as these sensitivity values may affect the normal values.

Specific normal values and comments that pertain to that particular nerve, or the referenced study, are also included. The normal values reported are taken from the articles referenced at the beginning of each nerve conduction technique. In order to use these normal values as standards, it is essential to follow each technique exactly as described. We present studies that use a standardized distance and document skin temperature. When these potential sources of error are not noted, it is so indicated.

Illustrations demonstrating the electrodiagnostic setup have been included to supplement the descriptions of nerve conduction technique. These are only intended to show the location of the active, reference, ground, and stimulating electrodes, as described in the text.

The contents are organized such that the manual begins with the cranial and cervical nerves, continues with nerves of the upper extremities (proximal to distal), and ends with nerves of the lower extremities (proximal to distal). There is no discussion of auditory or visual evoked responses, because measurement of these requires additional equipment that may not be present in many electrodiagnostic laboratories. It is our hope that this volume will be a practical and useful manual for those who perform clinical electrodiagnosis.

Joel A. DeLisa, M.D.
Keith Mackenzie, M.D.

Contents

Blink Responses Latency

General: Electrical stimulation of the supraorbital nerve elicits the blink reflex response which consists of two separate components: an early R1 and a late R2. Visual and auditory stimuli give a response with only one component. Whereas R1 is evoked only on the side of electrical stimulation, R2 is recorded bilaterally with unilateral electrical stimulation. The patient is positioned either in an armchair, relaxed and with the eyes half closed, or in a dark room with the eyes gently closed.

Pickup: The active surface electrode is placed on the belly of the orbicularis oculi below the canthus. To pick up consensual R2 on a second channel, a second pickup is attached to the opposite orbicularis oculi muscle. A second ground is not needed.

Reference: The reference is placed on the side of the nose.

Ground: The ground is placed on the forehead or cheek.

Stimulation: Electrical stimulation is applied over the supraorbital nerve, which is in the groove that is palpable at the medial third of the superior orbit, with the cathode placed over the supraorbital foramen. The infraorbital or mental nerve can be used instead of the supraorbital. Stimulation intensity

---

Kimura J, Powers JM, Van Allen MW: Reflex response of orbicularis oculi muscle to supraorbital nerve stimulation: Study in normal subjects and in peripheral facial paresis. *Arch Neurol* 21:193–199, 1969.

Kimura J, Giron LT, Young SM: Electrophysiological study of Bell palsy. Electrically elicited blink reflex in assessment of prognosis. *Arch Otolaryngol* 102:140–143, 1976.

Kimura J, Bodensteiner J, Yamada T: Electrically elicited blink reflex in normal neonates. *Arch Neurol* 34:246–249, 1977.

is usually approximately 3 to 8 mA (up to 16 to 20 mA) with duration of stimulus between 0.1 and 1 msec. Stimulus of low intensity causes the second response of the blink reflex to have a prolonged latency. Thus it is necessary to determine the stimulus intensity that will evoke the maximum R2 amplitude. With better stimulus control, there is less variability and more reproducibility of responses.

Electromyograph settings:

- Frequency—8 Hz to 8 kHz
- Sweep speed—5 msec/div (may need 10 msec/div if R2 latency is prolonged)
- Gain—50 to 100 μV/div
- Rate—not to be more than 1/sec (a faster rate may produce habituation)

Normal values: ($N = 83$ normal adult subjects, supraorbital nerve stimulation)

R1 usually is a biphasic or triphasic wave (occasionally polyphasic). It tends to habituate slowly and is a brief, relatively synchronous reflex.

R2 is polyphasic and habituates quickly with a decrease in amplitude and duration with repetitive stimulation. R2 correlates with clinically observed blink of the eyelids.

R1 component latency—10.6 ± 2.5 msec (mean ± 3 SD). In normals, the difference between values for R1 on each side is less than 1.2 msec. Since R1 appears only ipsilaterally, to compare right with left, both sides must be stimulated.

R2 component latency—Direct R2 (ipsilateral to the side of stimulus) is 31 ± 10 msec (mean ± 3 SD).

Consensual R2 latency (contralateral to the side of stimulus) is 32 ± 11 msec (mean ± 3 SD). The difference between values for R2 consensual and R2 direct is normally less than 5 msec (mean ± 3 SD). This measurement only requires "one" stimulus, since R2 appears ipsilaterally and contralaterally to the side stimulated.

Neonates: ($N = 30$)

R1 component latency—12.1 ± 0.96 msec (mean ± 1 SD).

R2 direct component latency—35.85 ± 2.45 (mean ± 1 SD). It was bilaterally absent in one-third and usually only ipsilateral in the other two-thirds.

Comments:

1. Latency is measured from the stimulus artifact to the initial deflection of the evoked potential (R1 or R2). Dr. Kimura suggests using the shortest latency of 8 stimulations.

2. Both R1 and R2 waves are probably due to a polysynaptic brainstem reflex, the blink reflex, with the afferent arc provided by the sensory branches of the trigeminal nerve and the efferent arc provided by the facial nerve motor fibers.

R1 is affected by lesions in:
- trigeminal nerve (afferent arc)
- pons (central arc)
- facial nerve (efferent arc)

R2 is affected by:
- level of consciousness
- habituation
- lateral medullary lesion
- contralateral hemispheric lesion
- parkinsonism
- medication [diazepam (Valium®)]

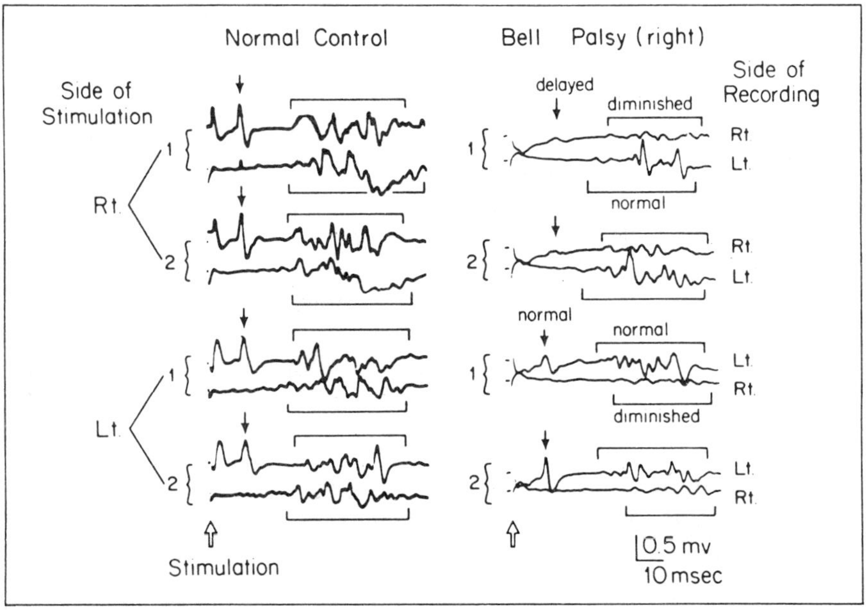

Figure 1 Two right-sided and two left-sided stimulations were delivered in each case to show consistency. In the patient, R_1 (*arrows*) and R_2 (*single brackets*) were delayed and small on the right side and normal on the left side regardless of side stimulated. This finding indicates a lesion involving efferent arc of reflex (facial nerve) on right side. (From Kimura, Giron, Young: *Arch Otolaryngol* 102:140–143, 1976. © 1976, American Medical Association.)

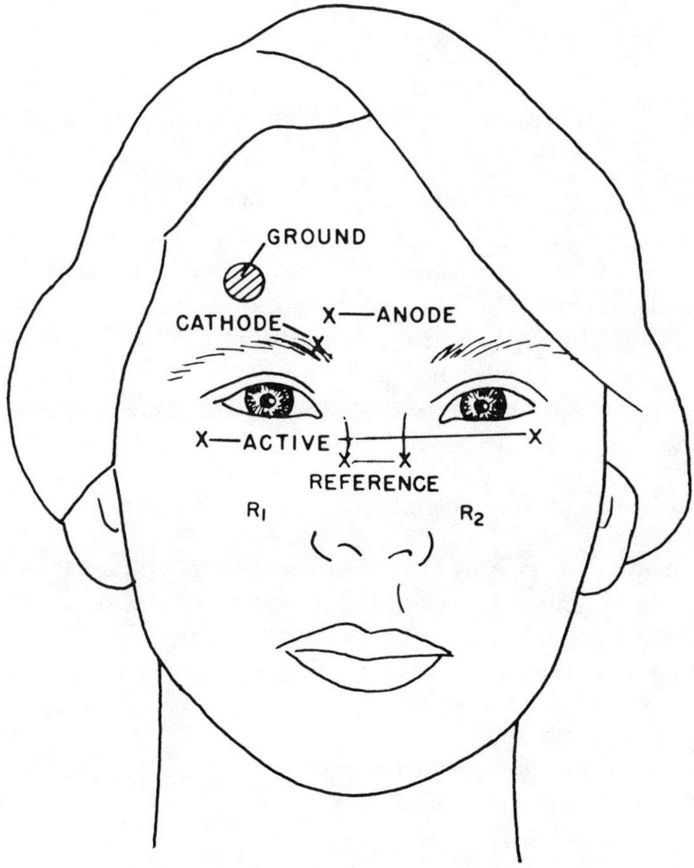

Figure 2 Blink responses latency.

Facial Nerve Distal Motor Latency

Pickup: The coaxial needle is placed in the orbicularis oris just superior to the corner of the mouth (a monopolar needle can be used in the same spot). Taylor et al. found that the coaxial needle gave a slightly better endpoint than the monopolar needle, although both gave satisfactory results. A surface electrode often did not give the desired sharp takeoff. If a monopolar needle is used, then a **reference** electrode is placed on the side of the nose.

Ground: The ground is placed on the contralateral forehead.

Stimulation: Waylonis and Johnson recommended that stimulation be applied just below the ear and anterior to the mastoid process (angle of the mandible). Taylor et al., however, suggested applying it directly over the stylomastoid foramen.

Electromyograph settings:

- Frequency—8 Hz to 8 kHz
- Sweep speed—2 msec/div
- Gain—250 μV

Waylonis GW, Johnson EW: Facial nerve conduction delay. *Arch Phys Med Rehabil* 45:539–547, 1964.

Taylor N, Jebsen RH, Tenckhoff HA: Facial nerve conduction latency in chronic renal insufficiency. *Arch Phys Med* 51:259–263, 1970.

Normal values: ($N = 78$)

Latency (to onset of the negative deflection of the evoked potential) according to Waylonis and Johnson:

Age	Mean (msec)	Range (msec)
Newborn–1 month	10.1	6.4–12.0
1 month–1 year	7.0	5.0–10.0
1–2 years	5.1	3.6–6.3
2–3 years	3.9	3.8–4.5
3–4 years	3.7	3.4–4.0
4–5 years	4.1	3.5–5.0
5–7 years	3.9	3.2–5.0
7–16 years	4.0	3.0–5.0

Waylonis and Johnson report normal values in adults as 3.4 ± 0.8 msec (mean $\pm$ 1 SD). Taylor et al. report normal values in adults as 4.0 ± 0.5 msec (mean $\pm$ 1 SD). Both measure from the stimulus artifact to the onset of the negative deflection of the evoked potential.

Comments: Temperature and distance were not reported in either of these studies. Evoked potential is often ragged and prolonged and does not necessarily indicate temporal dispersion.

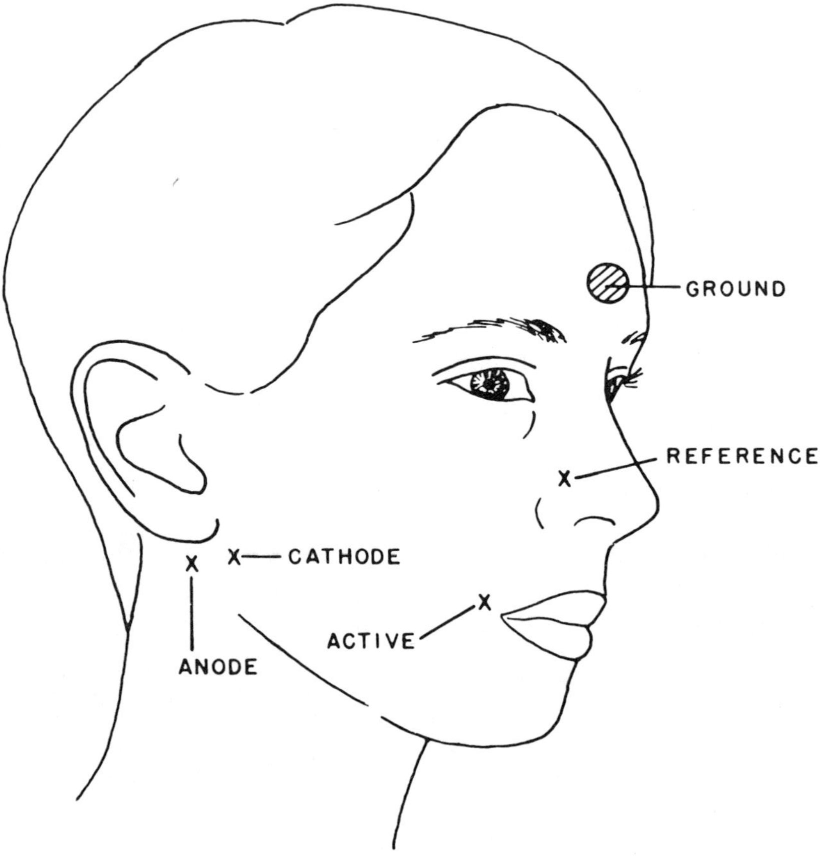

Figure 3 Facial nerve distal motor latency.

Spinal Accessory Nerve Motor Latency

Pickup: The active surface electrode is placed over the motor end plate of the upper trapezius muscle, approximately 5 cm lateral to the seventh cervical spinous process.

Reference: The reference is placed over a thoracic spinous process.

Ground: The ground is placed between the stimulus and the recording points.

Stimulation: The stimulation is applied about 1 to 2 cm posterior to the border of the sternocleidomastoid muscle at the level of the upper margin of the thyroid cartilage.

Electromyograph settings:

- Frequency—8 Hz to 8 kHz
- Sweep speed—2 msec/div
- Gain—500 μV

Normal values: ($N = 25$, ages 10 to 60)
Latency—1.8 to 3.0 msec

Comments: The temperature is not indicated. The distance between the stimulating and recording electrodes varied from 5.0 to 8.5 cm. The technique of measuring is not indicated, but probably represents a straight line.

Cherington M: Accessory nerve. Conduction studies. *Arch Neurol* 18:708–709, 1968.

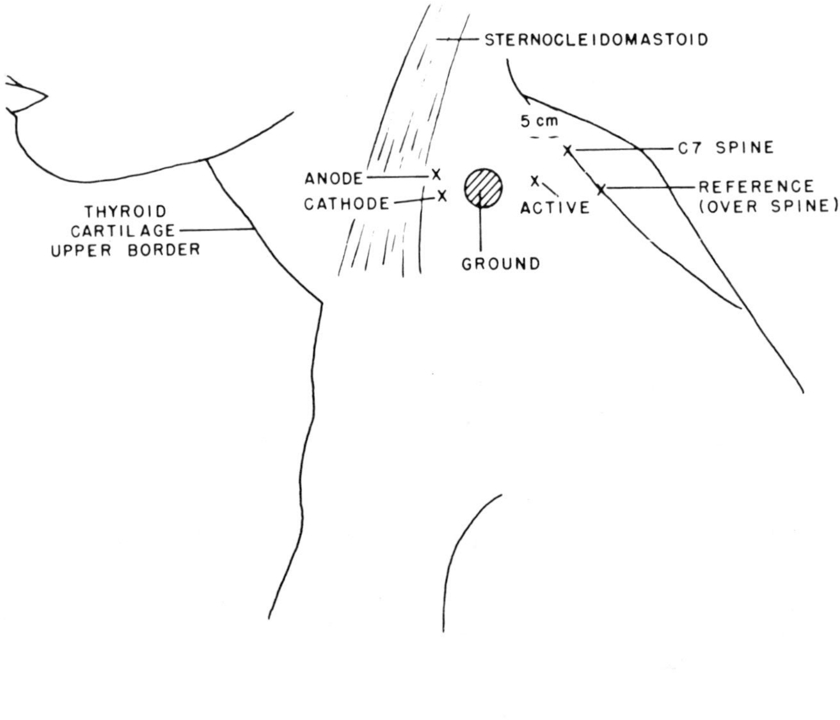

Figure 4 Spinal accessory nerve motor latency.

Phrenic Nerve Motor Latency

Pickup: The active surface electrode is placed in the eighth intercostal space in the anterior axillary line.

Reference: The reference is placed 3.5 to 5.0 cm from the active, either in the ninth intercostal space or posteriorly in the eighth intercostal space.

Ground: The ground is placed on the chest wall over the upper pectoral region.

Stimulation: Stimulation is applied at the posterior border of the sternocleidomastoid muscle at the level of the upper margin of the thyroid cartilage.

Electromyograph settings:

- Frequency—8 Hz to 8 kHz
- Sweep speed—5 msec/div
- Gain—250 μV

Normal values: ($N = 18$ normal adults, 4 were tested bilaterally)

Latency—7.7 ± 0.8 msec (mean ± 1 SD)

Amplitude—160 to 500 μV

Comments: Care must be taken to avoid concurrently stimulating the brachial plexus. Distance was not indicated, and temperature was apparently not measured.

Davis JN: Phrenic nerve conduction in man. *J Neurol Neurosurg Psychiatry* 30:420–426, 1967.

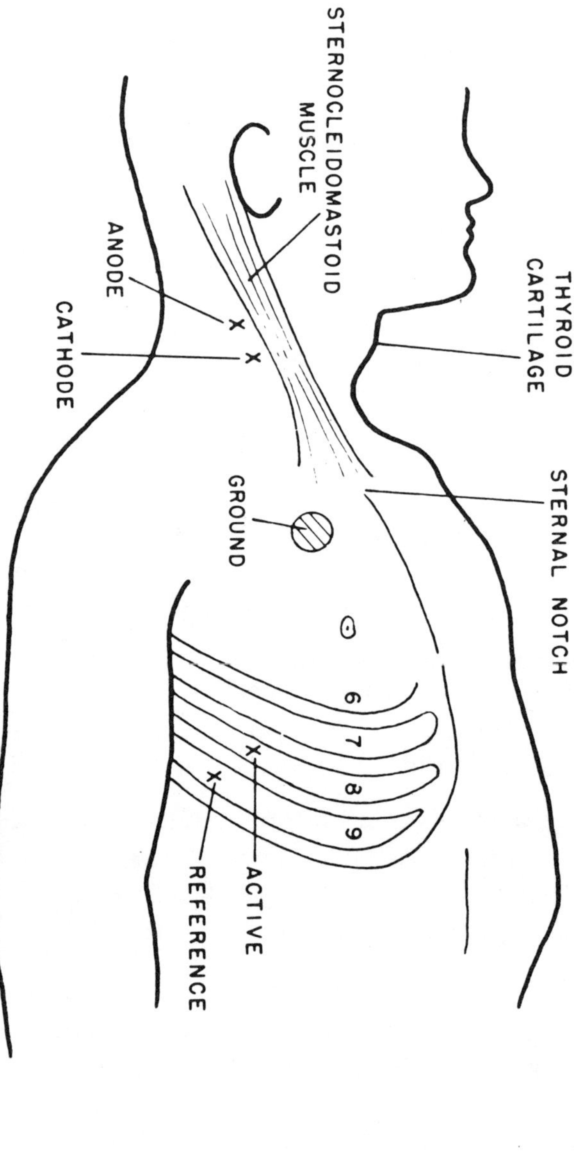

Figure 5 Phrenic nerve motor latency.

Long Thoracic Nerve Motor Latency

Pickup: The active surface electrode is a monopolar needle electrode placed into the digitation of the serratus anterior muscle at the fifth thoracic rib level in the midaxillary line.

Reference: The reference is placed 20 mm caudally to the active electrode.

Stimulation: The cathode of the surface stimulation electrode is placed at Erb's point (above the upper margin of the clavicle, lateral to the clavical head of the sternocleidomastoid muscle). The anode is located above and medially.

Electromyograph settings:

- Frequency—8 Hz to 8 kHz
- Sweep speed—5 msec/div
- Gain—500 μV

Distance: Distance is measured with obstetric calipers. The range of distance from the point of stimulation to the point of recording is 170 to 230 mm.

Normal values: ($N = 25$ normal adult subjects)
Latency—3.9 ± 0.6 msec (mean ± 1 SD)

Comments: No skin temperature was taken.

Kaplan PE: Electrodiagnostic confirmation of long thoracic nerve palsy. *J Neurol Neurosurg Psychiatry* 43:50–52, 1980.

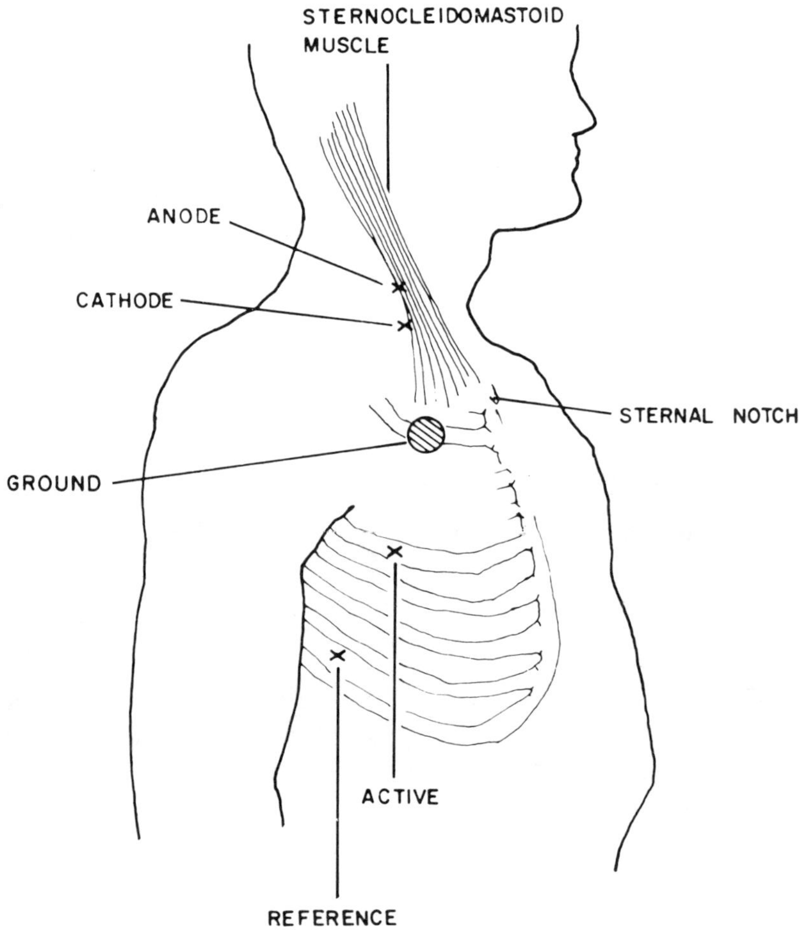

Figure 6 Long thoracic nerve motor latency.

Suprascapular Nerve Motor Latency to Supraspinatus and Infraspinatus

Stimulation: The cathode is slightly above the upper margin of the clavicle and lateral to the clavicular head of the sterno-cleidomastoid muscle. The anode is superior medially.

Electromyograph settings:

- Frequency—8 Hz to 8 kHz
- Sweep speed—2 msec/div
- Gain—500 μV

To supraspinatus ($N = 62$):

Pickup and reference: The coaxial needle is inserted medial to the midpoint of the scapular spine and just above the spine. It is inserted in a downward and forward direction until the scapula is touched, then the needle is withdrawn several millimeters. Shoulder abduction confirms the needle placement. The study is done with the patient sitting with arms at side.

Ground: The ground is placed between the stimulation and pickup sites.

Distance: A measuring tape is used with the arm at the side, and the range is 7.4 to 13.8 cm.

Normal values: Latency—2.7 ± 0.5 msec (mean ± 1 SD); normal range—1.7 to 3.7 msec. The M wave recorded with a coaxial needle electrode is polyphasic and of large amplitude.

Kraft GH: Axillary, musculocutaneous and suprascapular nerve latency studies. *Arch Phys Med Rehabil* 53:383–387, 1972.

To infraspinatus ($N = 62$):

Pickup and reference: The coaxial needle is inserted into the infraspinatus muscle several centimeters lateral to the medial border of the scapula and several centimeters below the scapular spine. It is inserted until it touches the scapular periosteum, and then withdrawn several millimeters. The study is done with the patient sitting with arms at side. External rotation of the shoulder confirms placement of the needle electrode.

Ground: The ground is placed between stimulation and pickup sites.

Distance: A measuring tape is used with arms at side, and the range is 15.0 to 19.5 cm. The distance is measured directly from the point of stimulation to the pickup using the shortest distance possible, rather than following the course of the nerve.

Normal value:

Latency—3.3 ± 0.5 msec (mean ± 1 SD); normal range—2.4 to 4.2 msec.

Comment: Studies were done in a room in which the temperature ranged from 75 to 84°F.

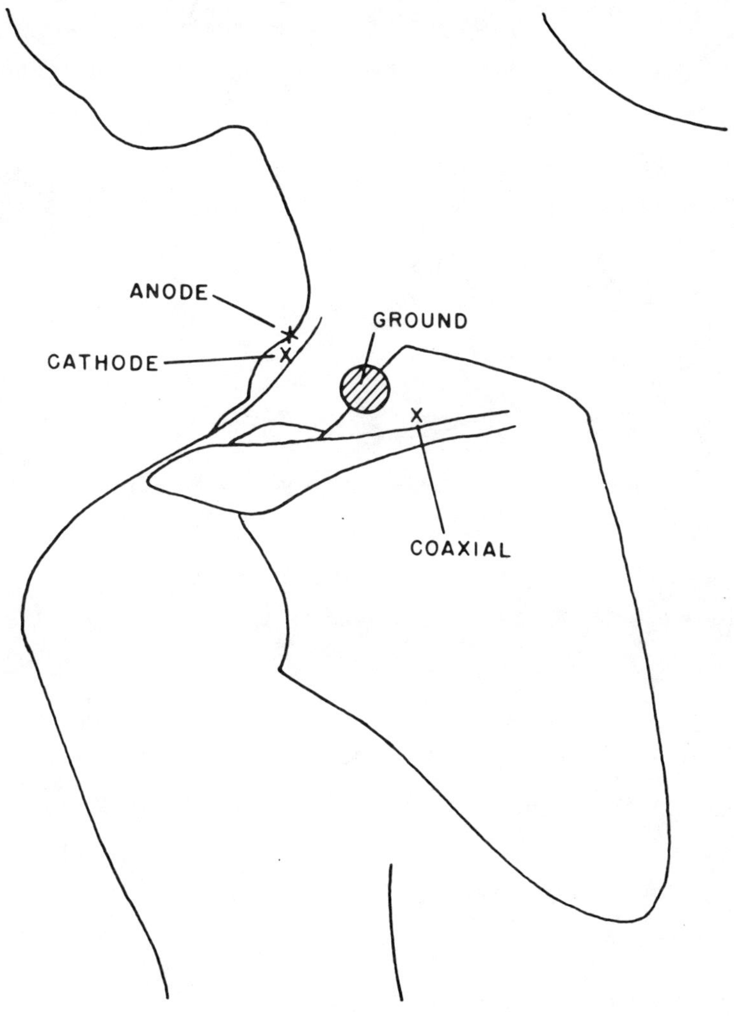

Figure 7 Suprascapular nerve motor latency to supraspinatus muscle.

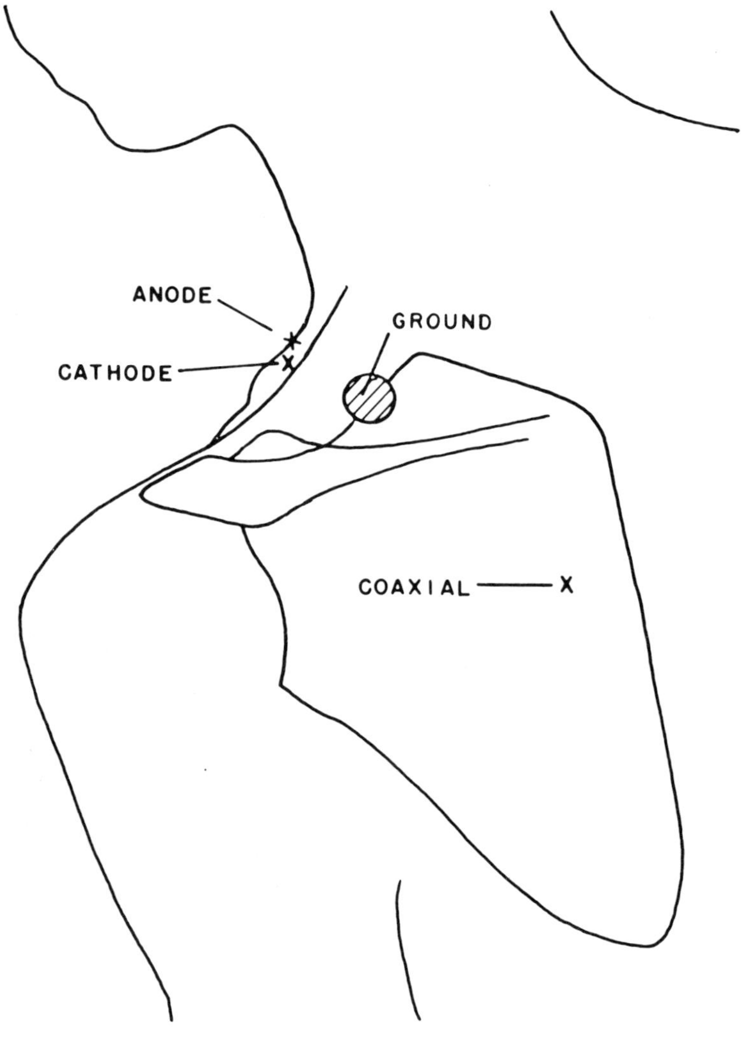

Figure 8 Suprascapular nerve motor latency to infraspinatus muscle.

Axillary Nerve Motor Latency to the Deltoid

Pickup: The active surface disc electrode (8 to 9 mm) is placed over the most prominent portion of the middle deltoid muscle, in the region containing the motor end plate band.

Reference: The reference is over the junction of the deltoid muscle and its tendon of insertion.

Ground: The ground is between the stimulating and pickup sites.

Stimulation: The cathode is placed slightly above the upper margin of the clavicle and lateral to the clavicular head of the sternocleidomastoid. The anode is superior medially.

Electromyograph settings:

- Frequency—8 Hz to 8 kHz
- Sweep speed—2 msec/div
- Gain—500 μV

Distance: Distance is measured using a flexible tape with the arm at the side, and ranges between 14.8 and 26.5 cm. Distance is measured from the point of stimulation directly to the pickup, taking the shortest distance possible, rather than following the course of the nerve.

Normal values: ($N = 62$)
Latency—3.9 ± 0.5 msec (mean ± 1 SD); normal range—2.8 to 5.0 msec.

Comments: Studies were done in a room in which the temperature ranged from 75 to 84°F.

Kraft GH: Axillary, musculocutaneous and suprascapular nerve latency studies. *Arch Phys Med Rehabil* 53:383–387, 1972.

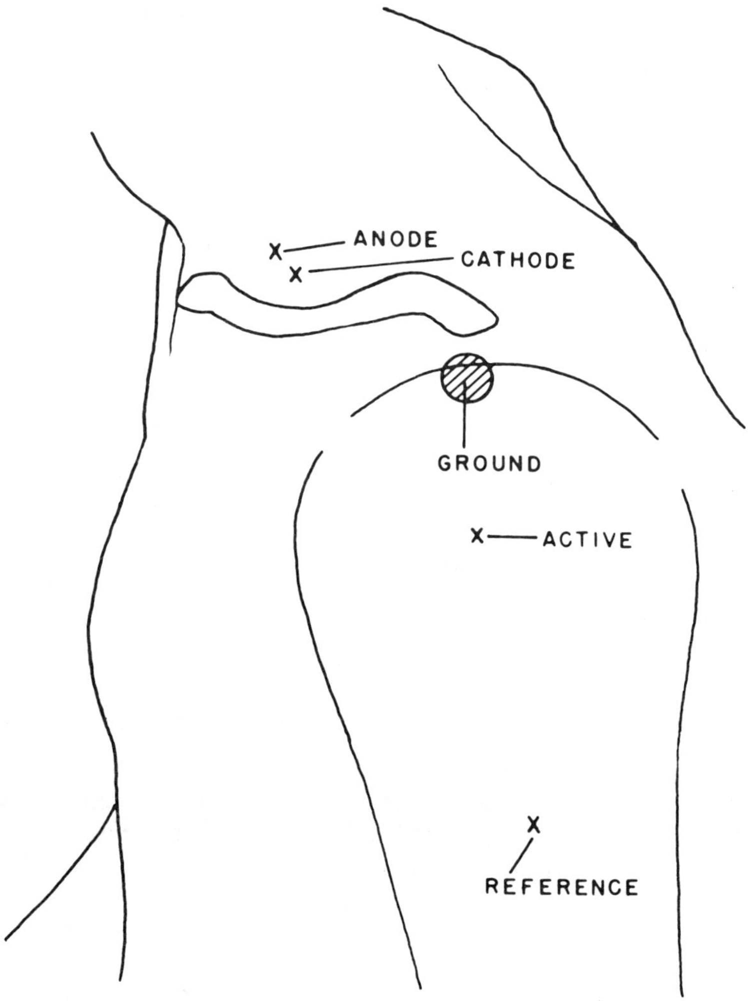

Figure 9 Axillary nerve motor latency to the middle deltoid muscle.

Musculocutaneous Motor Latency to the Biceps Brachii

Pickup: The active surface electrode is placed just distal to the midportion of the biceps brachii muscle.

Reference: The reference is placed proximal to the antecubital fossa, in the region of the junction of the muscle fibers and the biceps brachii tendon.

Ground: The ground is over the deltoid muscle.

Stimulation: The active cathode is slightly above the upper margin of the clavicle and lateral to the clavicular head of the sternocleidomastoid. The anode is superior medially.

Electromyograph settings:

- Frequency—8 Hz to 8 kHz
- Sweep speed—2 msec/div
- Gain—500 μV

Distance: When a measuring tape with the arm at the side is used, the range is 23.5 to 41.5 cm. Distance is measured from the point of stimulation directly to the pickup site, taking the shortest distance possible, rather than following the course of the nerve.

Normal value: ($N = 62$)
Latency—4.5 ± 0.6 msec (mean ± 1 SD); normal range—3.3 to 5.7 msec.

Comments: Studies were done in a room in which the temperature ranged from 75 to 84°F. The initial negative deflection of the evoked compound muscle action potential is less vertical and the amplitude generally lower than that seen in the axillary nerve motor latency to the deltoid muscle.

Kraft GH: Axillary, musculocutaneous and suprascapular nerve latency studies. *Arch Phys Med Rehabil* 53:383–387, 1972.

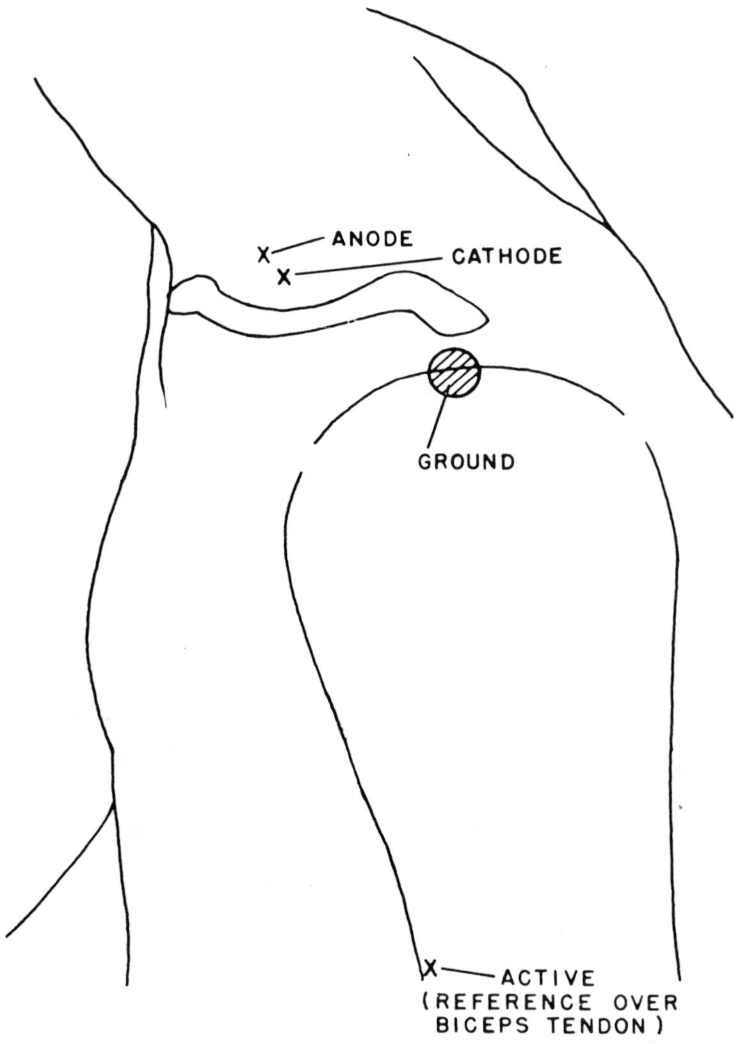

Figure 10 Musculocutaneous motor latency to the biceps brachii muscle.

Musculocutaneous Sensory Latency and Nerve Conduction Velocity

Pickup: The active surface electrode is placed over the anterior branch of the nerve. A line is drawn between the stimulating point and the radial artery at the wrist. The active electrode is placed along this line 12 cm from the cathode.

Reference: The reference is 4 cm distal.

Ground: The ground is placed between the points of stimulation and recording.

Stimulation: The cathode is at the elbow crease just lateral to the biceps tendon, and antidromic stimulation is used.

Electromyograph settings:

- Frequency—2 Hz to 2 kHz
- Sweep speed—2 msec/div
- Gain—10 μV

Normal values: (60 nerves in 30 normal adult subjects)

Latency to *onset* of the negative phase of the compound sensory nerve action potential—1.8 ± 0.1 msec (mean ± 1 SD); range—1.6 to 2.1 msec.

Latency to *peak* of the negative phase of the compound sensory nerve action potential—2.3 ± 0.1 msec (mean ± 1 SD); range—2.2 to 2.6 msec.

Spindler HA, Felsenthal G: Sensory conduction in the musculocutaneous nerve. *Arch Phys Med Rehabil* 59:20–23, 1978.

$$\text{Conduction velocity} = \frac{12 \text{ cm}}{\text{latency to onset in msec}}$$

$$= 65 \pm 3.6 \text{ msec (mean} \pm 1 \text{ SD)}$$

Amplitude—24 ± 7.2 μV (mean ± 1 SD); range—12 to 50 μV.

Right and left arm latency difference—<0.3 msec (mean ± 2 SD).

Comments: Temperature was not indicated, although all of the examinations were done at a room temperature of 23.9°C.

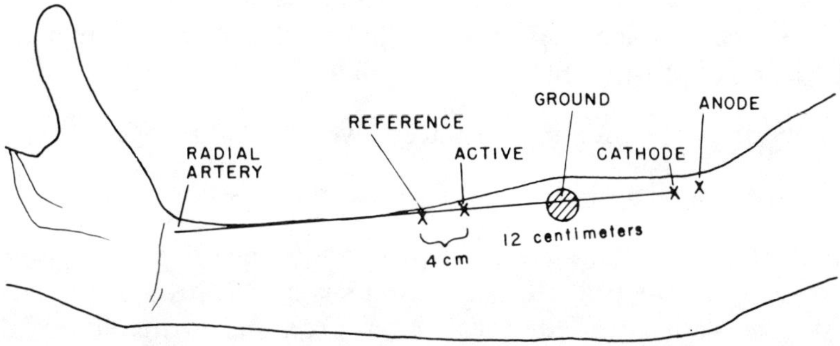

Figure 11 Musculocutaneous sensory latency and nerve conduction velocity (antidromic technique).

Radial Nerve Motor Nerve Conduction Velocity

Pickup: The active electrode is a monopolar needle inserted into the extensor indicis proprius muscle, which is located about two fingerbreadths proximal to the ulna styloid, just radial to the ulna at a depth of about 0.5 inch. Placement of the needle can be confirmed by extension of the second finger.

Reference: The reference is placed over the fifth finger.

Ground: The ground is between pickup and stimulation sites.

Stimulation: (Testing distal to proximal segments)

1. To test the branch to the extensor indicis proprius muscle, the nerve is stimulated 3 to 4 cm proximal to the site of the active electrode.

2. To test the forearm portion of the radial nerve, it is stimulated in the lateral antecubital space, approximately 5 to 6 cm proximal to the lateral epicondyle of the humerus, between the brachialis and brachioradialis muscles.

3. To test the upper arm segment of the radial nerve in the region of the spiral groove, the nerve is stimulated just posterior to the deltoid muscle insertion. (Note: If the nerve is deep, increased stimulus duration may be necessary).

Jebsen RH: Motor conduction velocity in proximal and distal segment of the radial nerve. *Arch Phys Med Rehabil* 47:597–602, 1966.

Trojaborg W, Sindrup EH: Motor and sensory conduction in different segments of the radial nerve in normal subjects. *J. Neurol Neurosurg Psychiatry* 32:354–359, 1969.

4. To test the entire radial nerve distal to Erb's point, it is stimulated in the supraclavicular fossa (at the angle of the clavicle and posterior aspect of the sternocleidomastoid muscle).

Distance: The distance is measured using a tape between the above elbow and forearm sites. An obstetrical caliper is used for a straight line measurement from Erb's point to the above elbow site. The arm is abducted 10°, the elbow flexed 10° to 15°, and the forearm pronated. The head is rotated away from the stimulation site.

Electromyograph settings:
- Frequency—8 Hz to 8 kHz
- Sweep speed—5 msec/div
- Gain—500 μV

Normal values: ($N = 49$)

Erb's point to above elbow—72 ± 6.3 m/sec (mean ± 1 SD), with a range of 56 to 93 m/sec.

Above elbow to the extensor indicis proprius—61.6 ± 5.9 m/sec (mean ± 1 SD), with a range of 48 to 75 m/sec.

Comments: No limb temperatures were measured.

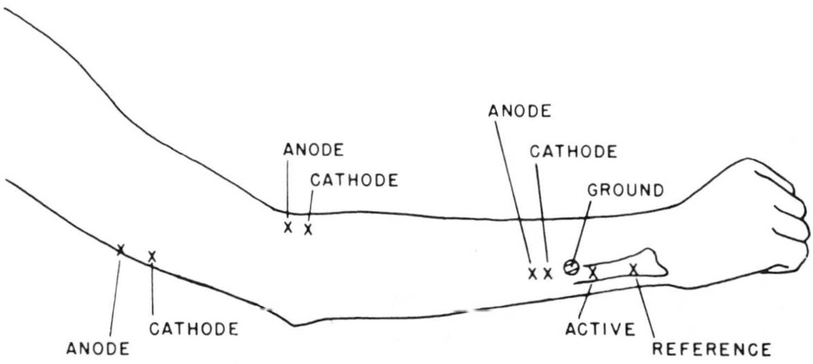

Figure 12 Radial nerve motor nerve conduction velocity.

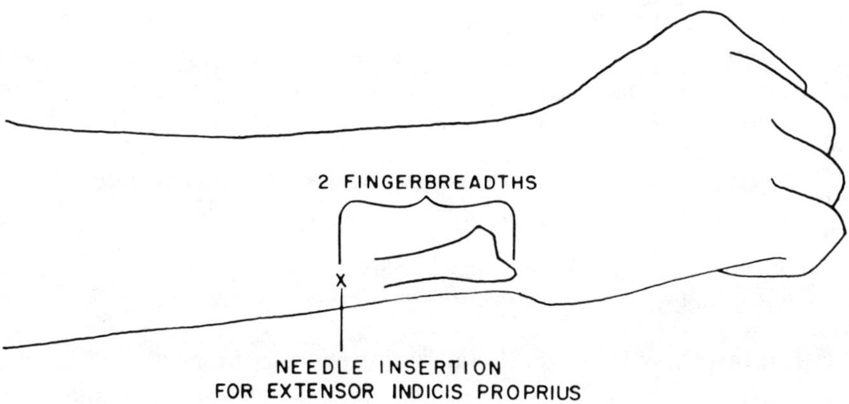

Figure 13 Needle electrode pickup in the extensor indicis proprius muscle for radial nerve motor nerve conduction velocity.

Radial Nerve Distal Sensory Latency

Pickup: The active surface electrode is placed over the major branch of the sensory nerve as it crosses the extensor pollicis longus tendon. The nerve crosses about 1 cm distal to the extensor retinaculum. It can be palpated over the tendon when the thumb is extended.

Reference: The reference is placed on the lateral side of the head of the second metacarpal.

Ground: The ground is placed between the stimulating site and the pickup.

Stimulation: The superficial radial nerve courses along the lateral border of the radius and can be palpated. Antidromic stimulation is applied at 10, 12, or 14 cm, with the cathode played distally. Distance is measured with the wrist neutral and the thumb lightly adducted.

Electromyograph settings:

- Frequency—8 Hz to 8 kHz
- Sweep speed—2 or 5 msec/div
- Gain—10 μV

Mackenzie K, DeLisa JA: Determining the distal sensory latency of the superficial radial nerve in normal adult subjects. *Arch Phys Med Rehabil* 62:31–34, 1981.

Normal values: (to peak of the negative phase of the compound sensory nerve action potential—$N = 49$)

Distance (cm)	2 msec/div (mean ± 2 SD)	5 msec/div (mean ± 2 SD)
10	2.3 ± 0.4 msec	2.4 ± 0.3 msec
12	2.6 ± 0.4 msec	2.8 ± 0.4 msec
14	2.9 ± 0.4 msec	3.1 ± 0.4 msec

Comments: Skin temperature was measured adjacent to the pickup electrode. The values reported are for a temperature range of 31 to 35°C. For colder hands, if the latency is outside the range of 2 SDs, hot packs are applied to warm them, and then the study repeated.

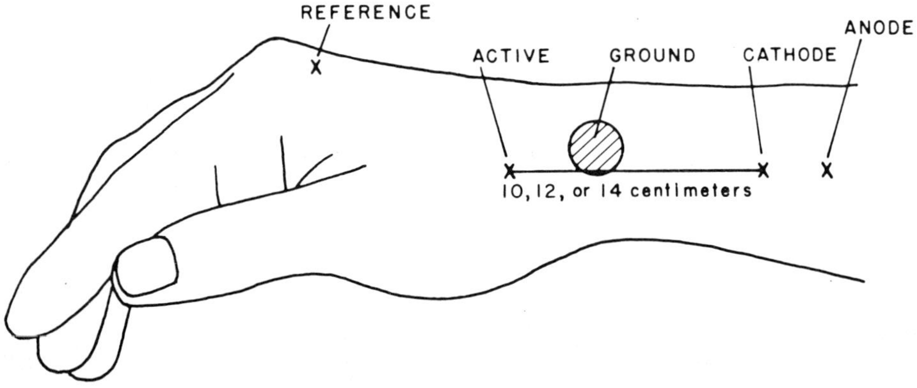

Figure 14 Radial nerve distal sensory latency (antidromic technique).

Median Nerve Motor Nerve Conduction Velocity and Latency

Pickup: The active surface electrode is placed one-half the distance (prominence of abductor pollicis brevis) between the metacarpophalangeal joint of the thumb and the midpoint of the distal wrist crease.

Reference: The reference is placed on the distal phalanx of the thumb.

Ground: The ground is between the pickup electrode and the stimulating electrode.

Stimulation: Stimulation is applied with the cathode 8 cm proximal to where the active electrode is placed, as shown in Fig. 15, between the flexor carpi radialis and the palmaris longus tendons. Proximal stimulation is applied in the medial aspect of the antecubital space, just lateral to the brachial artery.

Electromyograph settings:

- Frequency—8 Hz to 8 kHz
- Sweep speed—5 msec/div
- Gain—1,000 μV

Melvin JL, Harris DH, Johnson EW: Sensory and motor conduction velocities in the ulnar and median nerves. *Arch Phys Med Rehabil* 47:511–519, 1966.

Melvin JL, Schuchmann JA, Lanese RR: Diagnostic specificity of motor and sensory nerve conduction variables in the carpal tunnel syndrome. *Arch Phys Med Rehabil* 54:69–74, 1973.

Buchthal F: Electrophysiological findings in entrapment of the median nerve of wrist and elbow. *J Neurol Neurosurg Psychiatry* 37:340–360, 1974.

Normal values: ($N = 47$)

Distal latency—3.7 ± 0.3 msec (mean ± 1 SD); range—3.2 to 4.2 msec.

Velocity—56.7 ± 3.8 m/sec (mean ± 1 SD); range—50.0 to 67.3 m/sec.

Amplitude of the evoked potential at the wrist—13.2 mV ± 5.0 (mean ± 1 SD); range—5 to 25 mV.
Amplitude of the evoked potential at the elbow—13.5 mV ± 4.1 (mean ± 1 SD); range—5 to 23 mV.

Comments: Skin temperature was not recorded.

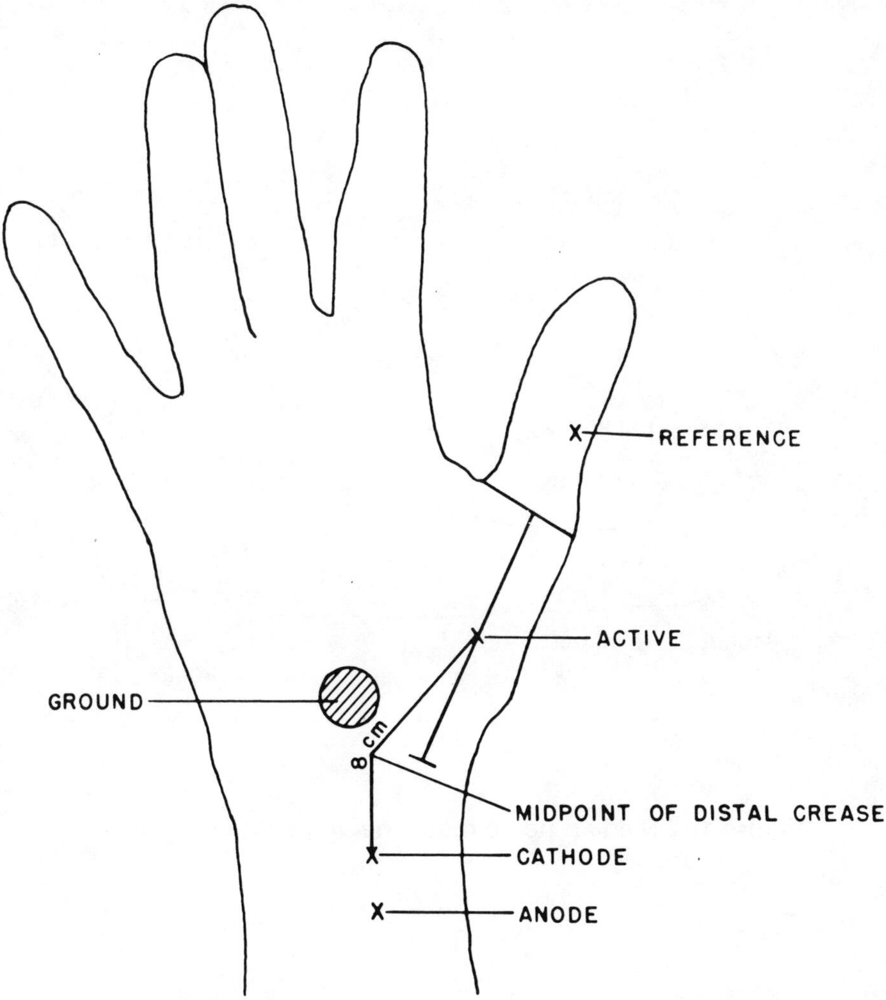

Figure 15 Median nerve distal motor latency.

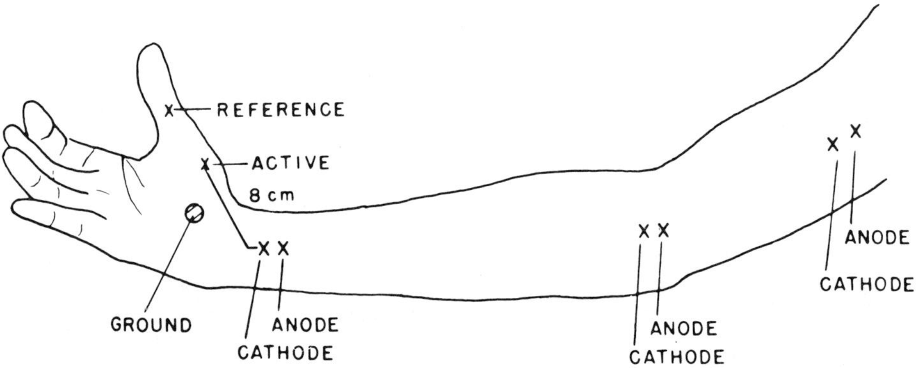

Figure 16 Median nerve motor nerve conduction velocity.

Median Nerve Distal Sensory Latency

ANTIDROMIC

Pickup: Ring recording electrodes are placed on digits 2, 3, or both. The active and reference electrodes are placed 4 cm apart, mounted in a plastic bar, with the active proximal at the base of the digits.

Ground: The ground is placed between the pickup and stimulation electrodes.

Stimulation: Stimulating cathode is applied 14 cm proximal (straight line) from the active ring electrode, over the median nerve between the tendons of the palmaris longus and flexor carpi ulnaris. Stimulation may also be applied medial to the biceps tendon. The anode is proximal.

ORTHODROMIC

Pickup: The active and reference electrodes are 4 cm apart mounted in a plastic bar with the active placed distally 14 cm from the cathode, over the median nerve between the tendons of the palmaris longus and flexor carpi radialis.

Ground: The ground is placed between the pickup and stimulating electrodes.

Melvin JL, Harris DH, Johnson EW: Sensory and motor conduction velocities in the ulnar and median nerves. *Arch Phys Med Rehabil* 47:511–519, 1966.

Johnson EW, Melvin JL: Sensory conduction studies of median and ulnar nerves. *Arch Phys Med Rehabil* 48:25–30, 1967.

Melvin JL, Schuchmann JA, Lanese RR: Diagnostic specificity of motor and sensory nerve conduction variables in the carpal tunnel syndrome. *Arch Phys Med Rehabil* 54:69–74, 1973.

Stimulation: Stimulation is applied with ring electrodes, 4 cm apart, around digits 2 and 3 with the cathode at the base of the digits.

Electromyograph settings:

- Frequency—8 Hz to 1.6 kHz
- Sweep speed—5 msec/div, measure on 2 msec/div
- Gain—10 μV

Normal values: ($N = 24$)

Latency to peak—3.2 ± 0.2 msec (mean ± 1 SD), for both the orthodromic and the antidromic techniques.

Forearm sensory conduction velocity—56.9 ± 4.0 m/sec (mean ± 1 SD); range—48 to 64.9 m/sec.

Amplitude of potentials—41.6 ± 25 μV (mean ± 1 SD); range—10 to 90 μV.

Comments: Skin temperature was not reported.

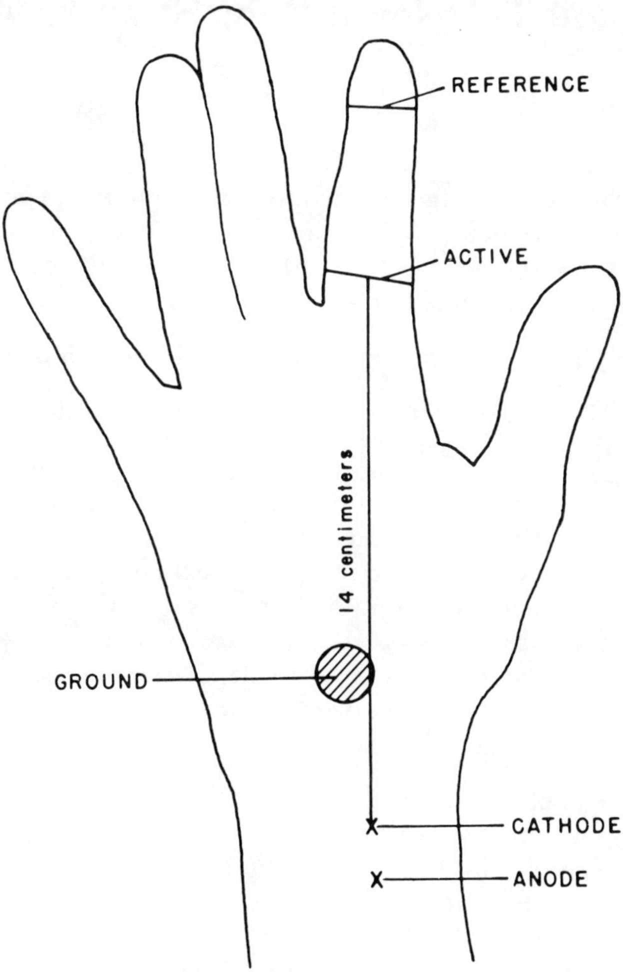

Figure 17 Median nerve distal sensory latency (palmar surface with antidromic technique).

C-8 and T-1 Nerve Root Stimulation

Pickup: The active surface electrode is placed in the hypothenar eminence (abductor digiti minimi) on a point midway between the distal wrist crease and the crease at the base of the fifth digit, at the junction of dorsal and palmar skin.

Reference: The reference is placed on the distal fifth digit.

Ground: The ground is over the lateral neck, back of the lateral neck, or over the back.

Stimulation: The active cathode is 1 to 2 cm lateral and slightly caudal to the seventh cervical spinous process. A 2-inch monopolar needle is inserted perpendicular to the skin surface in a sagittal plane until the tip rests directly over the vertebral transverse process. If the needle is not at this depth, the current intensity required to depolarize the nerve roots greatly increases. The anode is placed over the bony scapula, close to the stimulating electrode.

Electromyograph settings:

- Frequency—8 Hz to 8 kHz
- Sweep speed—3 msec/div is best for takeoff and 5 msec/div is best for entire M response
- Gain—500 μV
- Duration of stimulus—0.1 to 0.2 msec
- Stimulus intensity—approximately 100 to 150 V

MacLean IC: Nerve root stimulation to evaluate conduction across the brachial and lumbosacral plexus. Recent advances in clinical electromyography. *AAEE Third Annual Continuing Education Course* 51–55, Sept 1980.

Normal values: A 0.4-msec difference from side to side = 1 SD. A 1-msec difference between the sides is abnormal, but problems must be ruled out at the wrist and elbow.

Comments:

1. The *C-8 and T-1 roots* are used to measure across the lower trunk and medial cord of the brachial plexus.

2. The *C-5 and C-6 roots* can be stimulated together as a pair to measure the conduction across the upper trunk and lateral cord of the brachial plexus. The stimulating needle electrode is placed 1 to 2 cm lateral to the C-5 spinous process with the surface recording electrode over the middle of the biceps brachii muscle.

3. The posterior cord can be evaluated by stimulating the *C-6, C-7, and C-8 roots.* The stimulating cathode electrode is put between the sites for the C-5 and C-6 and the C-8 and T-1 stimulation. The surface recording electrode is over the middle of the triceps brachii muscle.

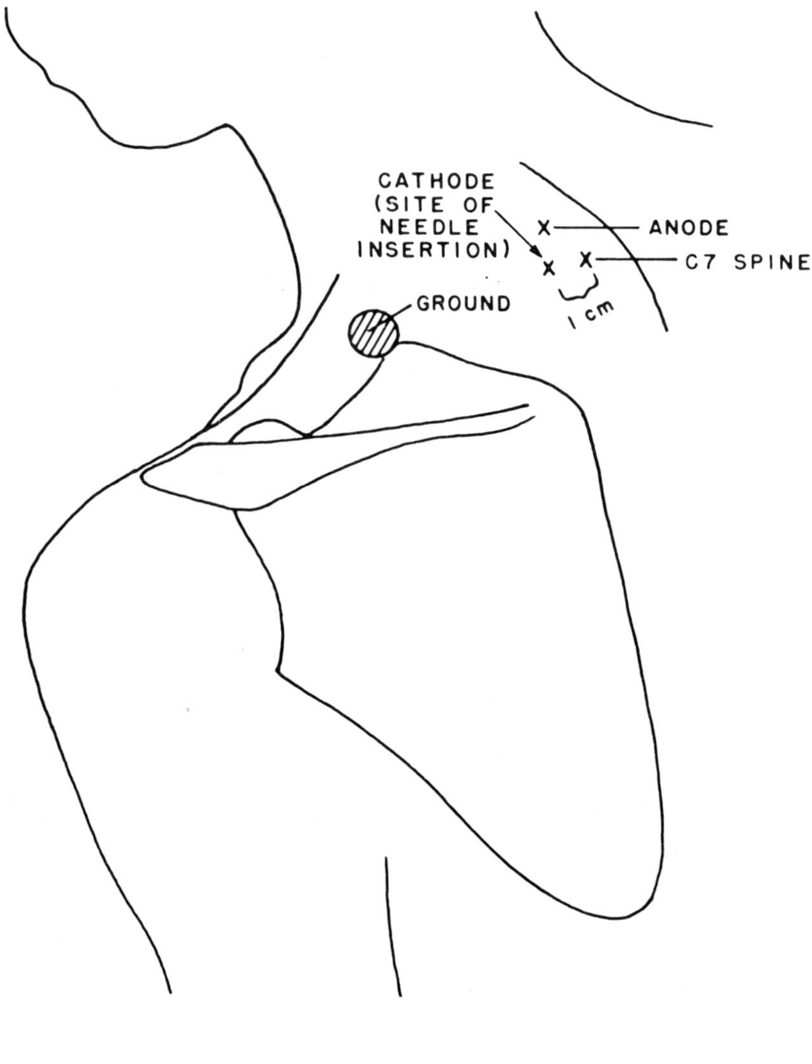

Figure 18 C-8 and T-1 nerve root stimulation.

Ulnar Nerve Motor Nerve Conduction Velocity

Pickup: The active surface electrode is placed on the abductor digiti minimi on a point midway between the distal wrist crease and the crease at the base of the fifth digit, at the junction of dorsal palmar skin.

Reference: The reference is on the fifth digit.

Ground: The ground is between the stimulation and pickup sites.

Stimulation: Stimulation is applied (a) 8 cm proximal to the active recording electrode and just over the flexor carpi ulnaris tendon, (b) just distal to the ulnar groove, and then (c) proximal to the ulnar groove.

Electromyograph settings:

- Frequency—8 Hz to 8 kHz
- Sweep speed—5 msec/div
- Gain—1,000 μV

Distance: Measurement across the elbow is done with the elbow flexed to 70° (elbow straight is 180°). The arm may be tested in the straight position and flexed for measurements.

Melvin JL, Harris DH, Johnson EW: Sensory and motor conduction velocities in the ulnar and median nerves. *Arch Phys Med Rehabil* 47:511–519, 1966.

Checkles, NS, Russakov AD, Piero DL: Ulnar nerve conduction velocity: Effect of elbow position on measurement. *Arch Phys Med Rehabil* 52:362–365, 1971.

Normal values: (*N* = 31 nerves in 18 adult subjects)

Distal latency to peak—3.2 ± 0.5 msec (mean ± 1 SD).

Motor forearm segment velocity—61.8 ± 5.0 m/sec (mean ± 1 SD); range—53 to 73 m/sec.

Motor across the elbow segment velocity—62.7 ± 5.5 m/sec (mean ± 1 SD); range—52 to 74 m/sec.

Amplitude of the evoked muscle response:

Stimulation site	Mean ± 1 SD mV	Range mV
Wrist	6.14 ± 1.90	2.34–9.94
Below elbow	5.60 ± 1.98	1.64–9.56
Across elbow	5.77 ± 1.79	2.19–9.35

Comments: The temperature was not recorded.

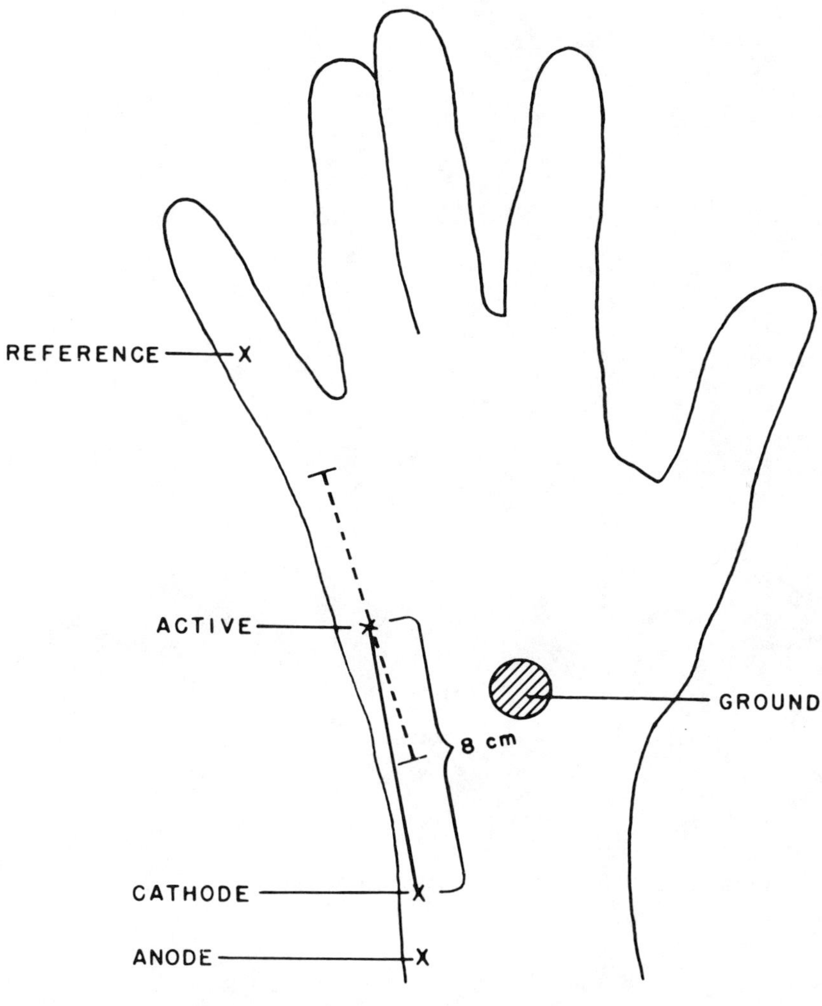

Figure 19 Ulnar nerve distal motor latency.

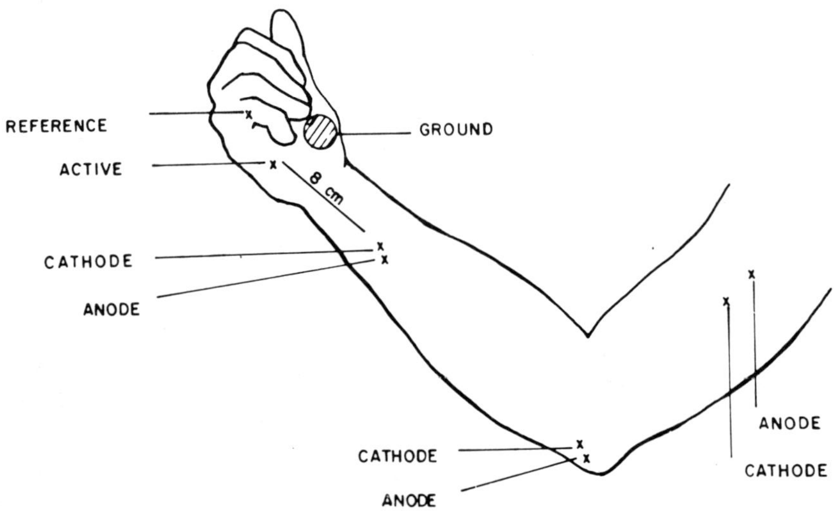

Figure 20 Ulnar nerve motor nerve conduction velocity.

Ulnar Nerve Distal Sensory Latency

ANTIDROMIC

Pickup: Ring active and reference electrodes are placed on the fifth digit with at least 4 cm separation, if possible. The active is proximal at the base of the digit.

Ground: The ground is between the stimulating and pickup electrodes.

Stimulation: Stimulation is applied 14 cm proximally, just radial to the flexor carpi ulnaris. The cathode is distal. Stimulation may also be applied proximally at the elbow in the ulnar groove.

ORTHODROMIC

Pickup: The active and reference electrodes are 4 cm apart with the active placed distally 14 cm from the cathode (over the flexor carpi ulnaris tendon).

Ground: The ground is placed between the stimulating and pickup electrodes.

Stimulation: Stimulation is applied with ring electrodes around the fourth and fifth fingers, 4 cm apart, with the cathode at the base of the digits.

Johnson EW, Melvin JL: Sensory conduction studies of median and ulnar nerves. *Arch Phys Med Rehabil* 48:25–30, 1967.

Electromyograph settings:

- Frequency—8 Hz to 1.6 kHz
- Sweep speed—5 msec/div initially; measure on 2 msec/div
- Gain—10 μV

Normal values: (N = 120)

Distal latency to peak—3.2 ± 0.25 msec (mean ± 1 SD), for both orthodromic and antidromic techniques.

Forearm sensory conduction velocity—57 ± 5.0 m/sec (mean ± 1 SD).

Amplitude of the potential—15 to 50 μV.

Comments: Skin temperature was not reported. With antidromic conduction the motor artifact may appear.

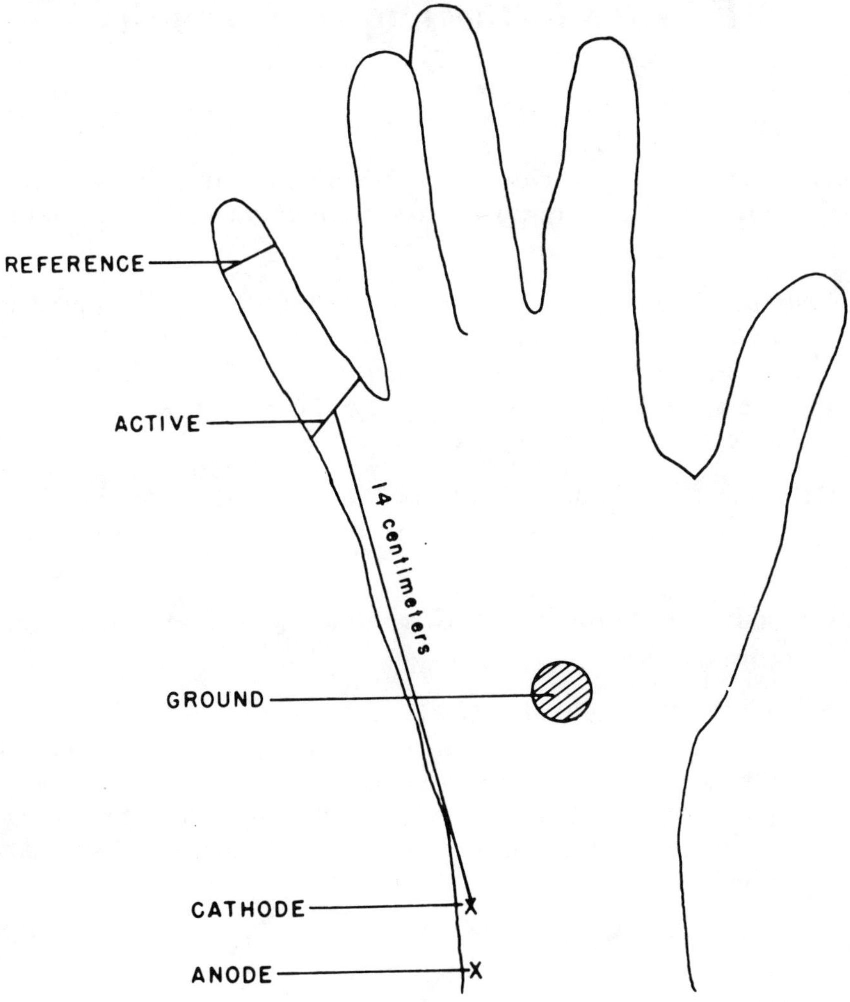

Figure 21 Ulnar nerve distal sensory latency (palmar surface with antidromic technique).

F Wave in the Upper Extremity

General: The F wave is not a reflex since the afferent and efferent arc of this response consist of the same alpha motor axon.

Pickup: The active surface electrode for the median nerve is over the abductor pollicis brevis. The active for the ulnar nerve is over the abductor digiti quinti. (This placement is the same as standard median or ulnar motor surface nerve placement; see pp. 33 and 43.)

Reference: For the median nerve, the reference is on the distal phalanx of the thumb; for the ulnar nerve, it is on the fifth digit.

Ground: The ground is between the stimulation and pickup sites.

Stimulation: Stimulation can be applied at the wrist, elbow, or in the axilla. However, axillary stimulation is difficult unless the collision technique is used (described in the above paper). Exact sites of stimulation are not described. *The stimulating electrode is distal and not proximal.* Supramaximal stimulation is used.

Electromyograph settings:

- Frequency—8 Hz to 8 kHz
- Sweep speed—5 msec/div
- Gain—250 μV

Kimura J: F-wave velocity in the central segment of the median and ulnar nerves. A study in normal subjects and in patients with Charcot-Marie-Tooth disease. *Neurology (Minneap)* 24:539–546, 1974.

Distance: The distance from the point of stimulus to the seventh cervical spine is measured as follows: surface measurements are made with subject in upright position and arm abducted to 90°. The hand is supinated for the median nerve and pronated for the ulnar nerve. Measurements are made along the course of the nerve to the axilla, then around the back of the shoulder (posteriorly) to the seventh cervical spinous process (T-1 is most prominent, seventh cervical is second most prominent).

Normal values: ($N = 33$)

Latency is measured to onset of the F wave and is the minimal latency after several trials (8 to 10 F waves).

Latency values (mean ± 1 SD msec)

Site	Median nerve	Ulnar nerve
Wrist	29.1 ± 2.3	30.5 ± 3.0
Elbow	24.8 ± 2.0	26.0 ± 1.8
Axilla	21.7 ± 2.8	21.9 ± 1.9

Latency difference between two stimulus points (mean ± 1 SD msec)

Site	Median nerve	Ulnar nerve
Elbow-wrist	4.3 ± 0.8	4.1 ± 0.8
Axilla-elbow	3.5 ± 0.5	4.1 ± 0.9

F wave velocity (m/sec)

$$= \frac{\text{(distance from stimulus point to C-7 spine)(2 mm)}}{\text{(F latency} - \text{M latency)} - 1 \text{ msec}}$$

F wave velocity

Median nerve	m/sec (mean ± 1 SD)
Wrist to spinal cord	59.2 ± 3.9
Elbow to spinal cord	62.2 ± 5.2
Axilla to spinal cord	64.3 ± 6.4

Ulnar nerve	m/sec (mean ± 1 SD)
Wrist to spinal cord	56.7 ± 2.9
Elbow to spinal cord	59.4 ± 4.7
Axilla to spinal cord	63.1 ± 5.9

Characteristics of F wave versus H wave and M wave:

1. In contrast with the H wave, the F wave can be recorded from almost every skeletal muscle in the adult. The latency of the F wave is longer with more distal sites of stimulation.

2. The amplitude of the F wave is usually less than that of the H wave.

3. Supramaximal stimulus, which abolishes the H wave, is used for recording F waves.

4. The F wave has a smaller amplitude than the M wave and is variable in latency and configuration when recorded with surface electrodes.

Comments: Latency values are not very useful until exact sites of stimulation are indicated and standards are established.

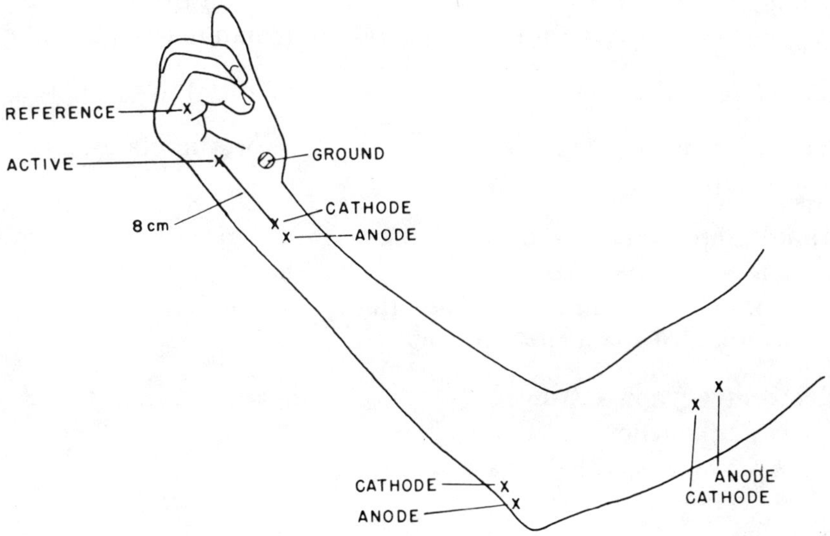

Figure 22 F wave in the upper extremity, testing the ulnar side.

Medial Antebrachial Cutaneous Nerve Conduction and Latency

Pickup: The active surface electrode is placed on the anteromedial surface of the forearm 9 to 12 cm from the cathode.

Reference: The reference is placed 3 to 4 cm distal to the active.

Ground: The ground is between the sites of stimulation and pickup.

Stimulation: The nerve is stimulated antidromically 2 to 4 cm lateral to the medial epicondyle of the humerus with the cathode located distally. This stimulation site is medial to the location of the median nerve.

Electromyograph settings:

- Frequency—8 Hz to 2 kHz
- Sweep speed—5 msec/div
- Gain—50 μV

Normal values: (N = 40)

NCV = 49.3 ± 3.8 m/sec (mean ± 1 SD)

Latency to the negative peak—1.7 to 2.6 msec (mean 2.1 msec)

Amplitudes—10 to 30 μV (mean 20 μV)

Comments: Skin temperature of the forearm was 31 to 33°C.

Pribyl R, You SB, Jantra P: Sensory nerve conduction velocity of the medial antebrachial cutaneous nerve. *Electromyogr Clin Neurophysiol* 19:41–46, 1979.

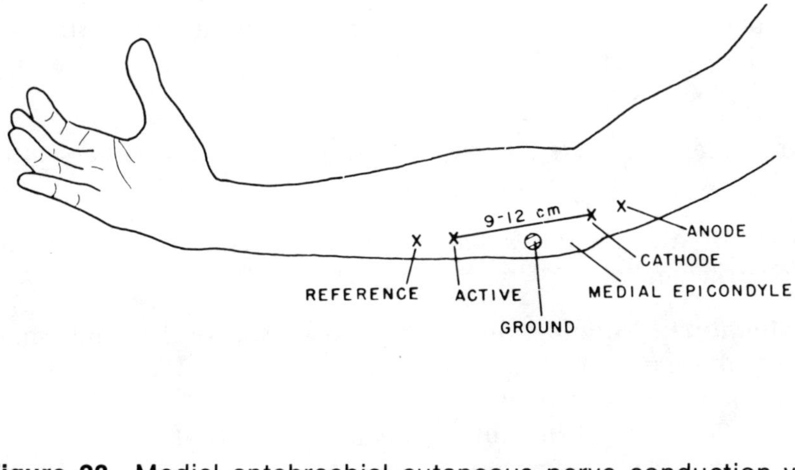

Figure 23 Medial antebrachial cutaneous nerve conduction velocity and latency (antidromic technique).

Bulbocavernosus Reflex Latency

Pickup: The active electrode is a coaxial needle inserted into the bulbocavernosus muscle. This muscle is superficial and is located under the scrotum on either side of the midline. Needle placement can be confirmed by squeezing the glans penis and observing the bulbocavernosus reflex. A monopolar needle can be inserted into the bulbocavernosus muscle.

Reference: The reference skin electrode is near the placement of the monopolar needle described above.

Ground: The ground is placed in a convenient location near the perineum.

Stimulation: Stimulation is on the dorsal side of the penile shaft and can be done using ring electrodes of a surface stimulator. The voltage required in this case usually is 50 to 200 V, or 5 to 20 mA, and the duration is 0.1 msec. Siroky et al. report using 0.5 msec duration.

Electromyograph settings:

- Frequency—8 Hz to 8 kHz
- Sweep speed—10 msec/div
- Gain—250 μV

Siroky MB, Sax DS, Krane RJ: Sacral signal tracing: The electrophysiology of the bulbocavernosus reflex. *J Urol* 122:661–664, 1979.

Dick HC, Bradley WE, Scott FB, Timm GW: Pudendal sexual reflexes. Electrophysiologic investigations. *Urology* 3:376–379, 1974.

Normal values:

Values were measured to the onset of the negative peak, which is often somewhat diffuse.

Siroky et al.—35 ± 2 msec (mean ± 1 SD); range—28 to 42 msec ($N = 52$ adult men).

Dick et al.—31 msec: average; range—24 to 40 msec ($N = 10$ adult men).

Comments: This study can also be done on women. Either the clitoris can be stimulated or a special stimulator can be attached to a Foley catheter and placed intraurethrally.

Several other investigators have also reported values. It appears that under 42 msec is normal with most techniques. However, Siroky's study defined abnormal as greater than 45 msec.

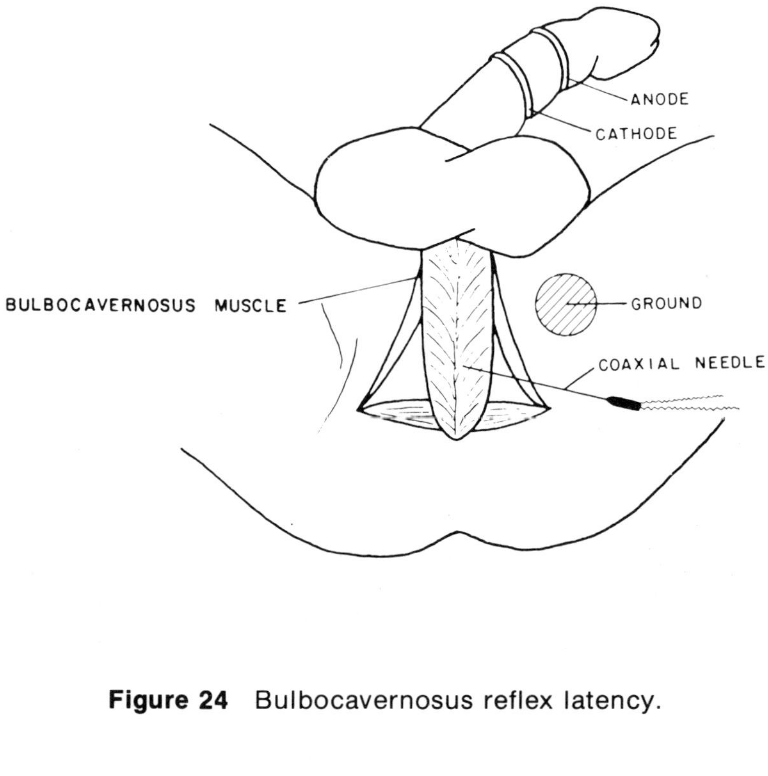

Figure 24 Bulbocavernosus reflex latency.

Lateral Femoral Cutaneous Latency and Nerve Conduction Velocity

ORTHODROMIC (Sarala et al.)

Pickup: The active surface disc electrode is placed 1 cm medial to the anterior superior iliac spine.

Reference: The reference is placed about 4 cm more cephalad.

Stimulation: Stimulation is applied using percutaneous bipolar stimulating electrodes placed 11 to 16 cm directly inferior to the anterior iliac spine on the anterior aspect of the thigh.

Electromyograph settings:

- Frequency—8 Hz to 1.6 kHz
- Sweep speed—5 msec/div
- Gain—10 μV

ANTIDROMIC (Butler et al.)

Pickup: Two strips of lead (1.2 × 1.9 cm) fixed in a plastic bar are placed 4 cm apart and 12 cm directly inferior to the anterior superior iliac spine on the anterior aspect of the thigh.

Stimulation: A 3-inch monopolar needle with a disc anode, or a bipolar needle, can be used. The needle is inserted above the inguinal ligament about 1 cm medial to the anterior superior iliac spine. The nerve is fairly superficial, and the depth of insertion is influenced by the degree of subcutaneous tissue.

Butler ET, Johnson EW, Kaye ZA: Normal conduction velocity in the lateral femoral cutaneous nerve. *Arch Phys Med Rehabil* 55:31–32, 1974.

Sarala PK, Nishihara T, Oh SJ: Meralgia paresthetica—Electrophysiologic study. *Arch Phys Med Rehabil* 60:30–31, 1979.

Normal values:

$$\text{Velocity} = \frac{\text{distance}}{\text{latency to negative peak}}$$

= 57.5 ± 8.61 m/sec (mean ± 2 SD)
Range—45.0 to 68.2 m/sec (Sarala et al.; $N = 20$ normal adults)

= 47.9 ± 3.7 m/sec (mean ± 2 SD)
Range—43 to 55 m/sec (Butler et al.; $N = 24$ normal adults)

Latency—1.8 to 3.1 msec over 12 to 16 cm (Sarala et al.); for 12 cm—2.6 ± 0.2 msec (mean ± 1 SD) (Butler et al.) Range—2.3 to 3.1 msec.

Amplitude of the nerve potential—10 to 25 μV (Butler et al.)

Comments: Skin temperature of the thigh ranged from 31.0 to 34.7°C in the study of Sarala et al. An averager (using 32 to 64 stimuli) was necessary in that study, as the amplitude of the nerve potential was 2 to 10 μV.

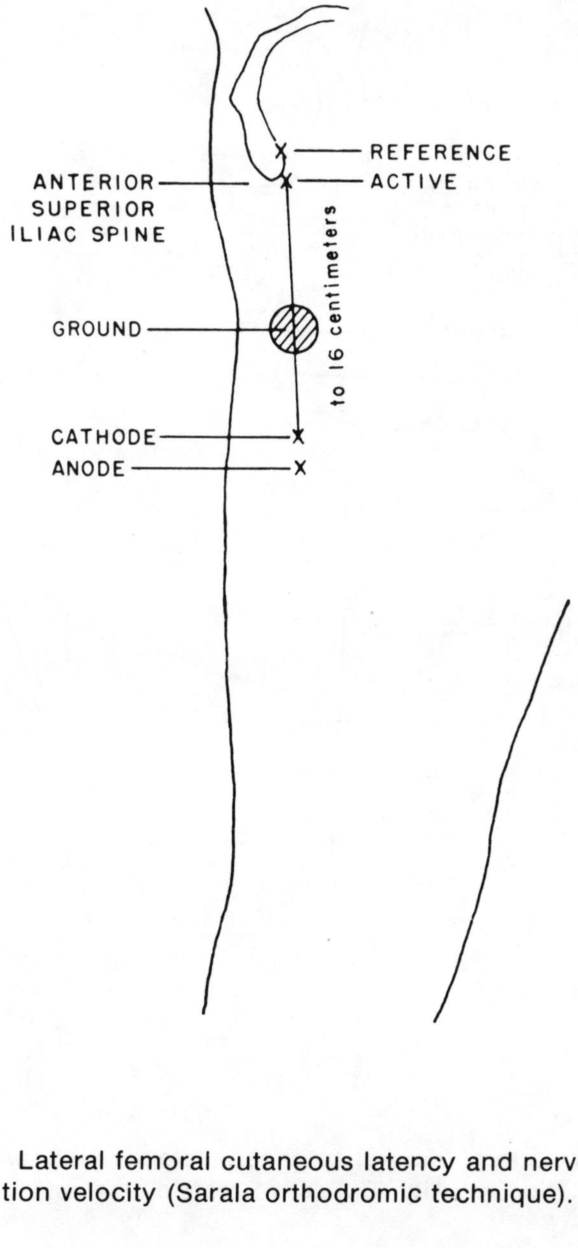

Figure 25 Lateral femoral cutaneous latency and nerve conduction velocity (Sarala orthodromic technique).

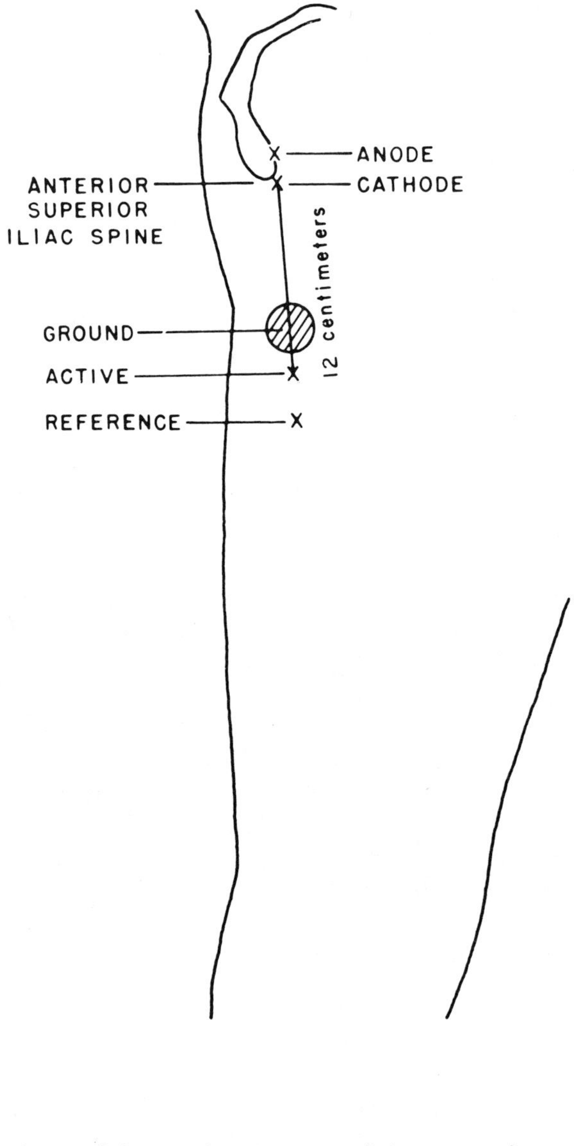

Figure 26 Lateral femoral cutaneous latency and nerve conduction velocity (Butler antidromic technique).

Femoral Nerve Motor Latency and Nerve Conduction Velocity

GASSEL

Pickup: Active—concentric needles are used for pickup. (A monopolar needle and surface electrode give similar results.) No difference was noted between placement in rectus femoris, vastus medialis, or vastus lateralis muscles if distance from stimulation was kept constant. Specific values are reported for 14 and 30 cm, although the table in Fig. 28 can be used for other distances.

Ground: The ground is between the stimulation and pickup sites.

Stimulation: Stimulation is applied just below the inguinal ligament and lateral to the femoral artery. Usually surface electrodes are used, but occasionally a monopolar needle is needed for stimulation.

Electromyograph settings:

- Frequency—8 Hz to 8 kHz
- Sweep speed—5 msec/div
- Gain—500 μV

Gassell MM: A study of femoral nerve conduction time. *Arch Neurol* 9:607–614, 1963.

Johnson EW, Wood PK, Power JJ: Femoral nerve conduction studies. *Arch Phys Med Rehabil* 49:528–532, 1968.

Normal values: ($N = 42$)

Latency (14 cm)—3.7 ± 0.1 msec (SD = 0.45 msec); range of distance—13 to 15 cm.

Latency (30 cm)—6.0 ± 0.15 msec (SD = 0.6 msec); range of distance—29 to 31 cm.

Mean conduction velocity calculated between 14 and 30 cm points—70 m/sec ± 7.8%.

JOHNSON et al.

Pickup: Surface pickups are used, with the active surface electrode over the "center" of the vastus medialis muscle. The mean distance from above the inguinal ligament to the pickup is 35.4 ± 1.9 cm.

Reference: The reference is over the patellar ligament.

Ground: The ground is between the stimulation and pickup sites.

Stimulation: Stimulation is applied just above the inguinal ligament and lateral to the femoral artery, in addition to below the ligament. The distance across the inguinal ligament is 5.5 cm, SD = 1.6 cm. Needle electrode tends to facilitate the technique.

Normal values: (N = 100 adults)

Above the inguinal ligament latency—7.1 ± 0.7 msec (mean ± 1 SD); range—6.1 to 8.4 msec.

Below the inguinal ligament latency—6.0 ± 0.7 msec (mean ± 1 SD); range—5.5 to 7.5 msec.

Delay across the inguinal ligament—1.1 ± 0.4 msec (mean ± 1 SD); range—0.8 to 1.8 msec.

Conduction velocity in the segment of nerve from above the inguinal ligament to the point of distal stimulation—66.7 ± 7.4 m/sec; range—50 to 96 m/sec).

Conduction velocity of the segment of the nerve from below the inguinal ligament to the distal point of stimulation—69.4 ± 9.2 m/sec; range—50 to 90 m/sec.

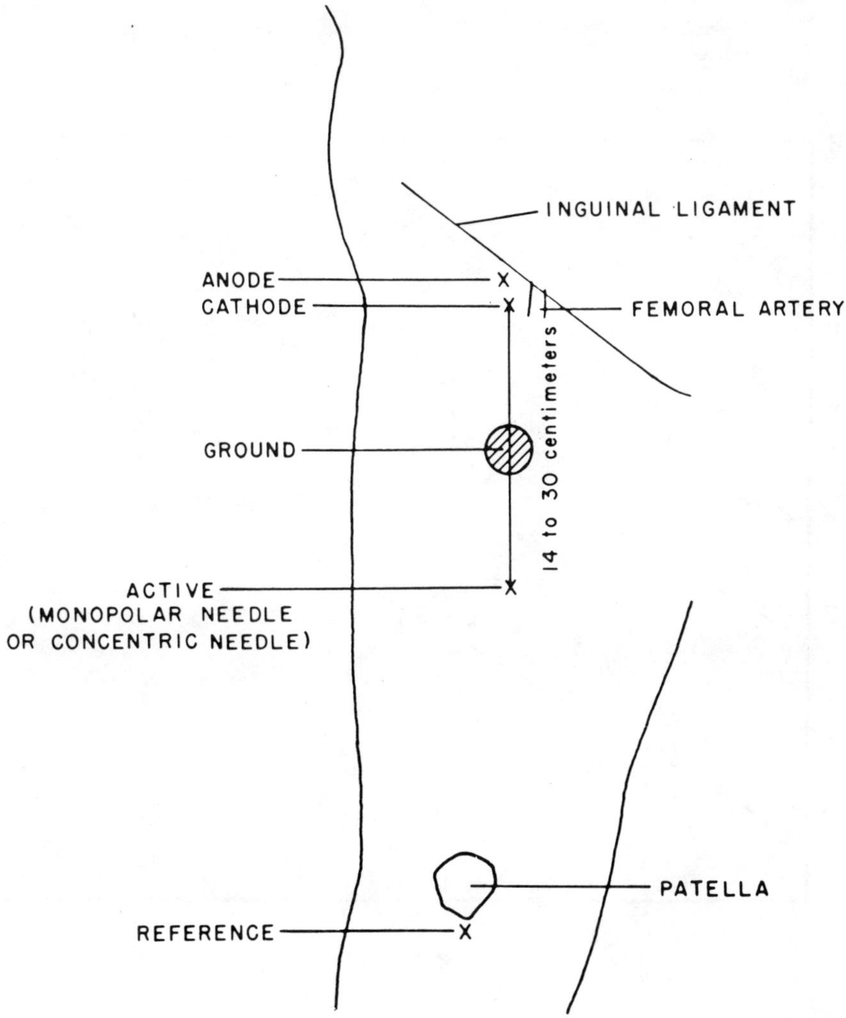

Figure 27 Femoral nerve motor latency and nerve conduction velocity (Gassel technique).

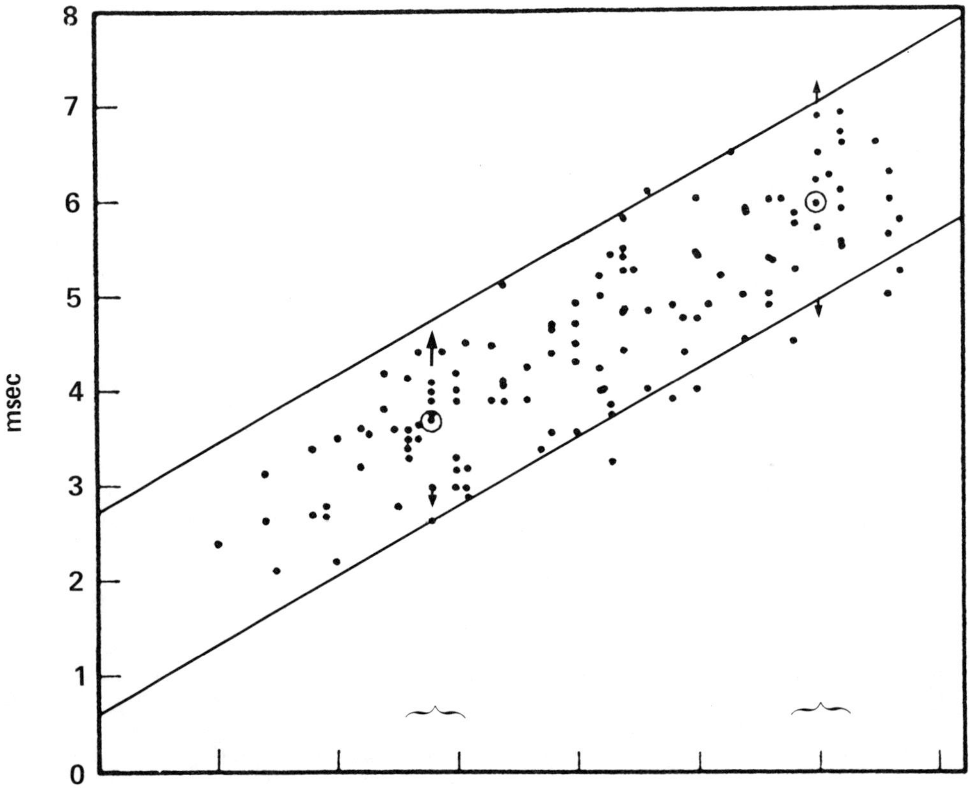

Figure 28 Femoral latency values by distance from the stimulating electrode. (From Gassell MM: *Arch Neurol* 9:607–614, 1963. © 1963, American Medical Association.)

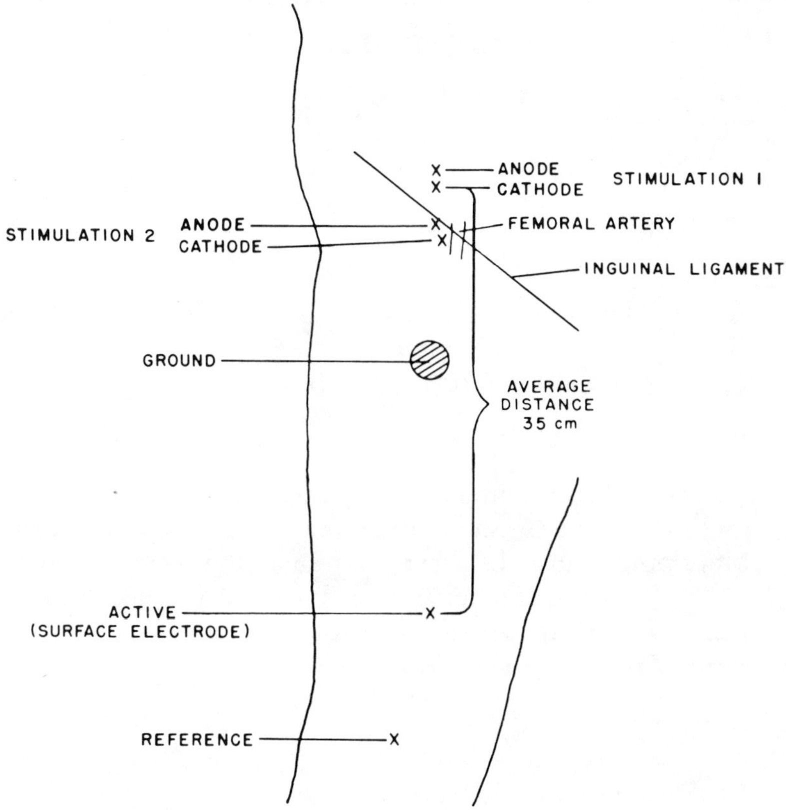

Figure 29 Femoral nerve motor latency and nerve conduction velocity (Johnson technique).

Peroneal Nerve to Extensor Digitorum Brevis Motor Nerve Conduction Velocity and Latency

Pickup: The active surface electrode is placed over the extensor digitorum brevis (EDB) muscle in the anterior lateral aspect of the proximal midtarsal area.

Reference: The reference is placed on the fifth toe.

Stimulation: Distal stimulation is applied about 8 cm proximal to the pickup, just lateral to the tibialis anterior tendon. More proximally, the nerve is stimulated just below the head of the fibula as the nerve curves around the bone. Finally, stimulation is applied in the popliteal space over the lateral third of the flexor skin crease.

Electromyograph settings:

- Frequency—8 Hz to 8 kHz
- Sweep speed—5 msec/div
- Gain—1,000 μV

Checkles NS, Bailey JA, Johnson EW: Tape and caliper surface measurements in determination of peroneal nerve conduction velocity. *Arch Phys Med Rehabil* 50:214–218, 1969.

Jimenez, J, Easton JK, Redford JB: Conduction studies of the anterior and posterior tibial nerves. *Arch Phys Med Rehabil* 51:164–169, 1970.

Normal values:

Distal latency if 8 cm used—4.5 ± 0.8 msec (mean ± 1 SD).

Below fibula head to ankle—

Checkles et al.: 1. Tape measure (length 31.6 ± 3.4 cm)
49.9 ± 5.9 m/sec (mean ± 1 SD)
Range—41.6 to 64.6 m/sec
($N = 32$)
2. Calipers (length 31.3 ± 3.3 cm)
49.4 ± 5.8 m/sec (mean ± 1 SD)
Range—41.2 to 64.0 m/sec

Jimenez et al.: **right:** 51.6 ± 4.1 m/sec (mean ± 1 SD); range—37 to 62 m/sec
left: 51.6 ± 3.5 m/sec (mean ± 1 SD); range—42 to 63 m/sec
($N = 39$).

Across fibular head—

Checkles et al.: 1. Tape measure (length 39.2 ± 3.1 cm)
51.1 ± 6.3 m/sec (mean ± 1 SD)
Range—41.6 to 62.7 m/sec
2. Calipers (length 38 ± 3.0 cm)
49.5 ± 6.1 m/sec (mean ± 1 SD)
Range—40.2 to 61.8 m/sec

Jimenez et al.: **right:** 53.9 ± 4.3 m/sec (mean ± 1 SD); range—42.3 to 63.7 m/sec
left: 52.80 ± 4.6 m/sec (mean ± 1 SD); range—44.1 to 65.3 m/sec

Comments: Anomalous innervation to the EDB occurs one-fifth of the time and is indicated by a different (smaller) wave shape when stimulating distally (partial anomaly) or by an absence of a wave potential (complete anomaly). The accessory peroneal nerve courses posterior and under the lateral malleolus, where stimulation is applied. The paper of Checkles et al. does not report temperatures. In the study of Jimenez et al. skin temperature in the forefoot was 29 to 34°C.

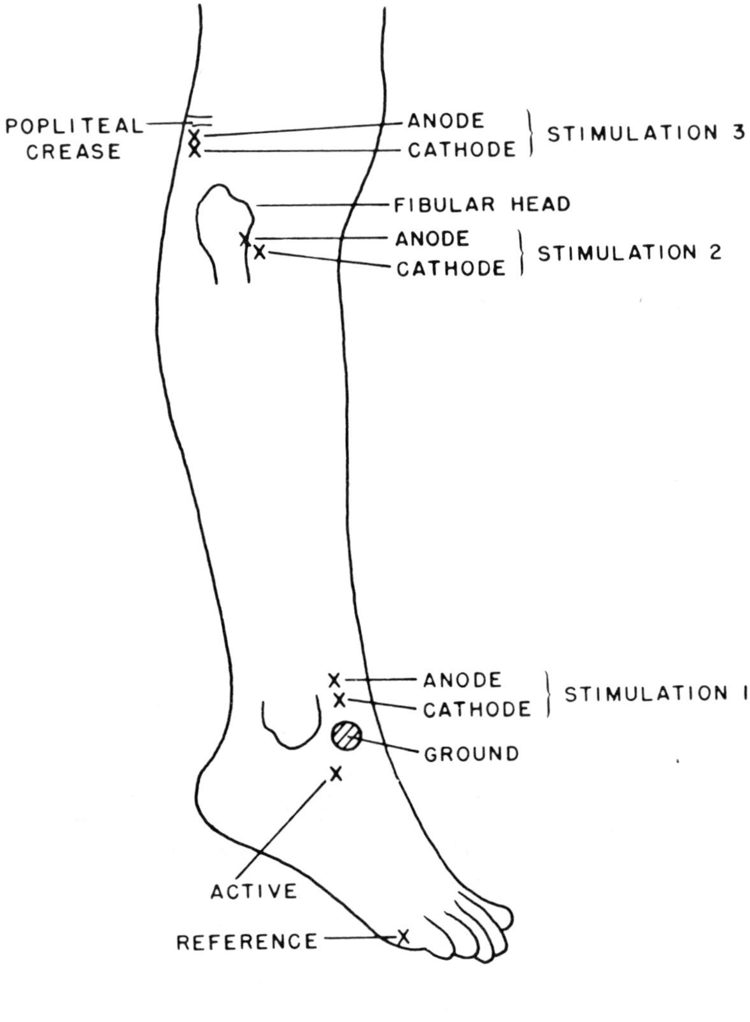

Figure 30 Peroneal nerve motor nerve conduction velocity to extensor digitorum brevis.

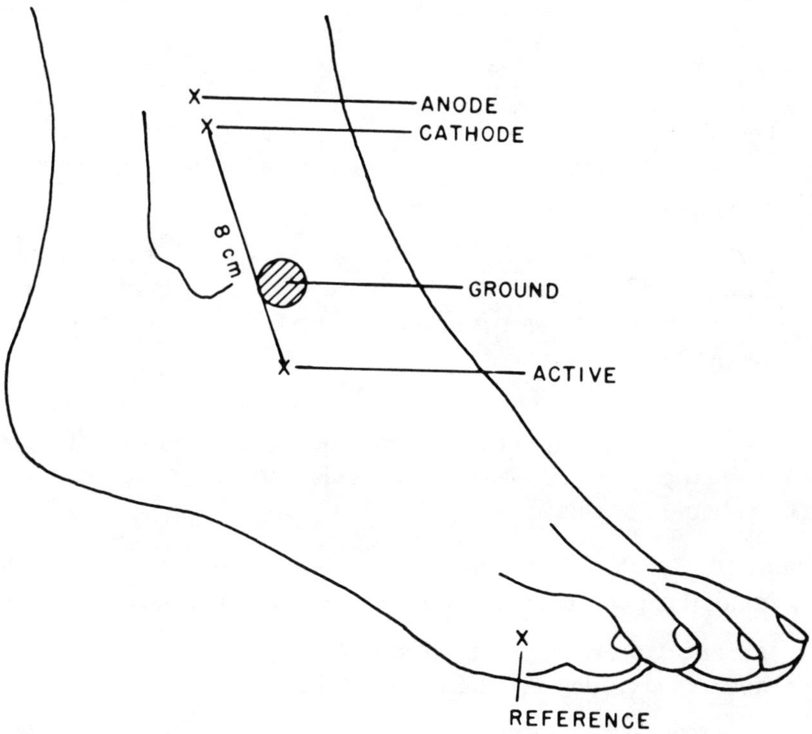

Figure 31 Peroneal nerve motor distal latency to the extensor digitorum brevis muscle.

Peroneal Nerve Conduction Velocity to Tibialis Anterior and Peroneus Brevis

Pickup: The active electrode was 32 mm (size of a TECA ground). Similar values are achieved using standard surface electrodes.

Tibialis anterior—The active surface electrode is placed at the junction of the upper third and lower two-thirds of a line between the tibial tuberosity and the tip of the lateral malleolus of the fibula.

Peroneus brevis—The active surface electrode is placed at the junction of the upper two-fifths and the lower three-fifths of a line between the head of the fibula and the tip of the lateral malleolus of the fibula.

Reference: *Tibialis anterior*—The reference is placed over the medial aspect of the tibia, 4 cm distal to the active electrode.

Peroneus brevis—The reference is placed 4 cm distal to the active electrode over the muscle tendon.

Ground: The ground is between the site of stimulation and the site of pickup.

Stimulation: Stimulation is applied above the head of the fibula and below the head of the fibula with approximately 10 cm between the two points of stimulation.

Devi S, Lovelace RE, Duarte N: Proximal peroneal nerve conduction velocity: Recording from anterior tibial and peroneus brevis muscles. *Ann Neurol* 2:116–119, 1977.

Electromyograph settings:

- Frequency—8 Hz to 8 kHz
- Sweep speed—2 msec/div
- Gain—250 μV

Normal values: (N = 34)

Latencies: (mean ± 1 SD)

	Above fibular head	Below fibular head
To tibialis anterior	4.7 ± 0.5 msec	3.0 ± 0.6 msec
Range	3.4–6.0 msec	2.0–4.4 msec
To peroneus brevis	5.0 ± 0.8 msec	3.0 ± 0.8 msec
Range	3.8–7.2 msec	1.7–5.4 msec

Nerve conduction velocity across fibular head:

To tibialis anterior—66.3 ± 12.9 m/sec (mean ± 1 SD)
To peroneus brevis—55.3 ± 10.2 m/sec (mean ± 1 SD)

Comments: Distances from point of stimulus to pickup were not specified. Skin temperature was also not specified. However, the room was kept at a constant temperature of 22.2 to 23.3°C.

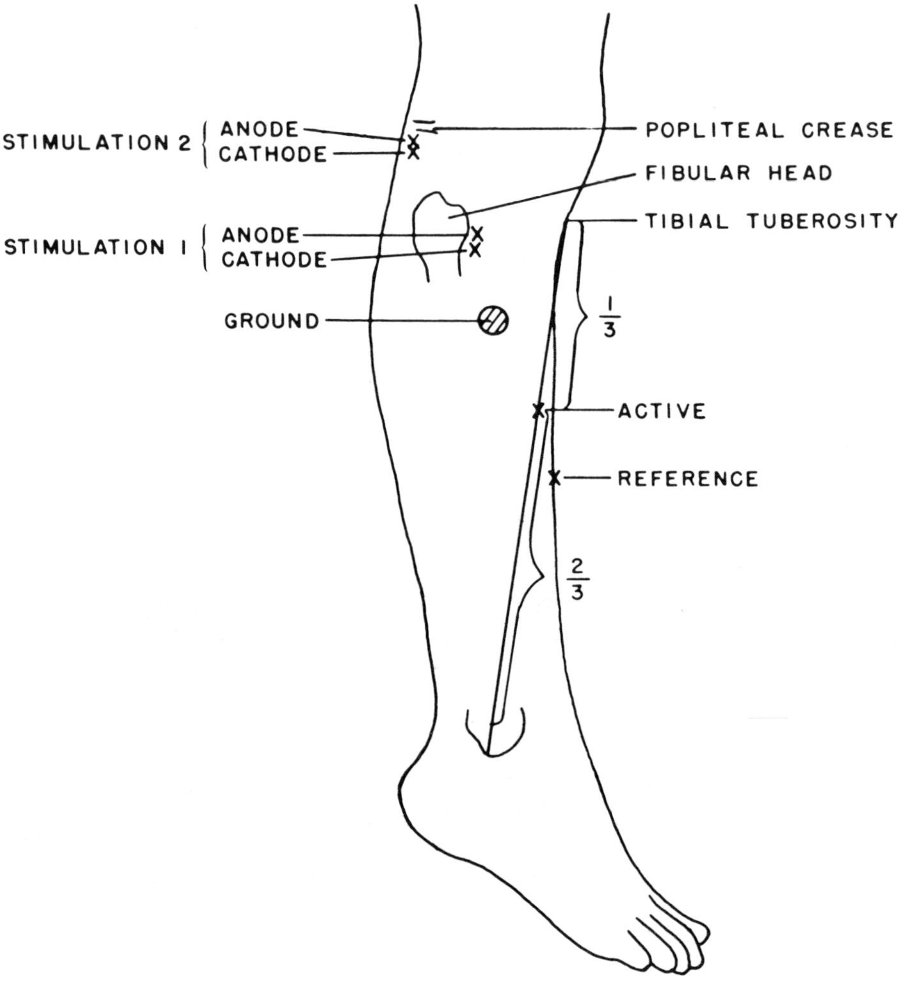

Figure 32 Peroneal motor nerve conduction velocity to tibialis anterior muscle.

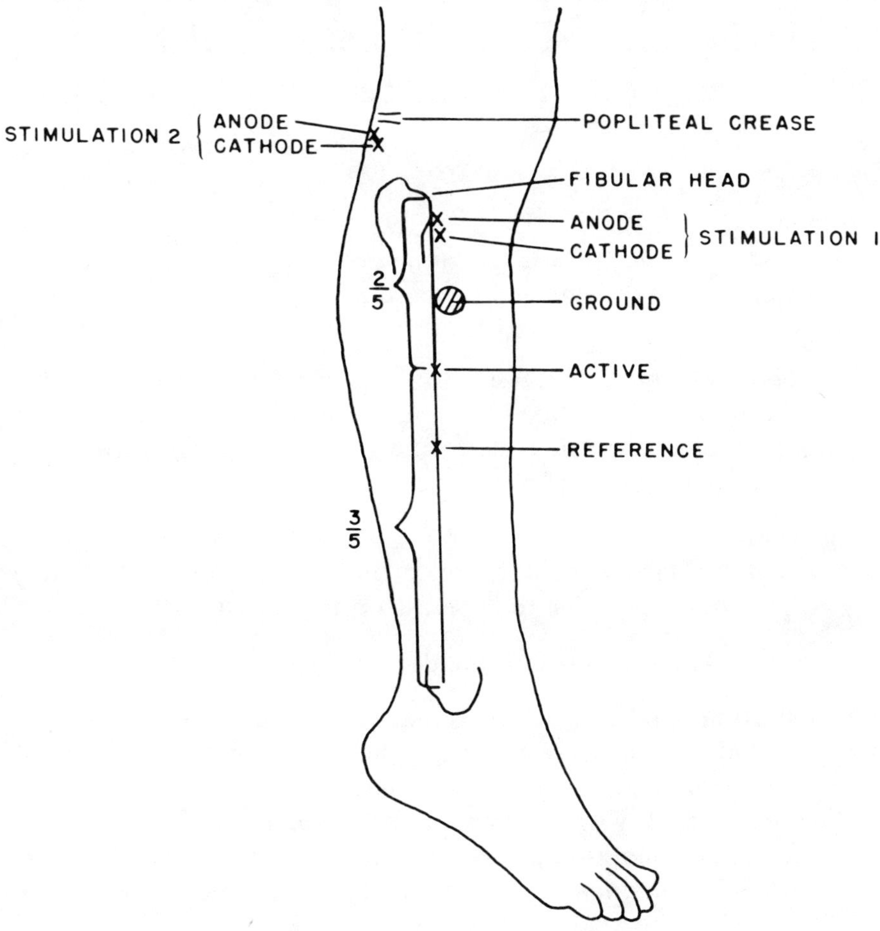

Figure 33 Peroneal motor nerve conduction velocity to peroneus brevis muscle.

Tibial Nerve Motor Nerve Conduction Velocity and Medial Plantar and Lateral Plantar Latencies

Pickup:

Medial plantar: The active surface electrode is 1 cm behind and 1 cm below the navicular tubercle (medial side of foot). Recording is from the abductor hallucis muscle.

Lateral plantar: The active surface electrode is directly below the lateral malleolus, bisecting the distance from the tip of the malleolus to the sole of the foot. Recording is from the abductor digiti minimi muscle.

Reference:

Medial plantar: The reference is on the large toe.
Lateral plantar: The reference is on the little toe.

Ground: The ground is on the dorsum of the foot.

Stimulation: *Distal distance* is measured from the pickup of the **medial plantar nerve** following the course of the nerve 1 cm posterior to the medial malleolus. Distances of 8 or 10 cm can be used, with the stimulation occurring posterior to the medial malleolus and above the flexor retinaculum. The *same site of stimulation* is used for the **lateral plantar nerve.** Measurements are made both with calipers and with a flexible tape measure for the medial plantar nerve segments. The ankle is in the neutral position (90°).

Fu R, DeLisa JA, Kraft GH: Motor nerve latencies through the tarsal tunnel in normal adult subjects: Standard determinations corrected for temperature and distance. *Arch Phys Med Rehabil* 61:243–248, 1980.

Jimenez J, Easton JK, Redford JB: Conduction studies of the anterior and posterior tibial nerves. *Arch Phys Med Rehabil* 51:164–169, 1970.

Proximal distance is measured at the crease of the popliteal fossa, at about the junction of the lateral third and medial two-thirds. Care must be taken not to stimulate too laterally, which stimulates the peroneal nerve instead.

Electromyograph settings:

- Frequency—8 Hz to 8 kHz
- Sweep speed—5 msec/div
- Gain—500 μV

Normal values: (N = 37 adults; no temperature correction, and using flexible tape measurements)

	8 cm (mean ± 1 SD)	10 cm (mean ± 1 SD)
Medial plantar latency:	3.4 ± 0.5 msec	3.8 ± 0.5 msec
Lateral plantar latency:	3.6 ± 0.5 msec	3.9 ± 0.5 msec

Motor NCV: 54.9 ± 7.6 m/sec (mean ± 1 SD)—Fu et al.
51.2 ± 3.9 m/sec (mean ± 1 SD)—Jimenez et al.

Comments: Skin temperature was measured below the medial malleolus, and the temperature range was 29 to 34°C (mean—32.1 ± 1.4°C). The article of Fu et al. has a table of temperature corrections, as well as values obtained using calipers instead of flexible tape.

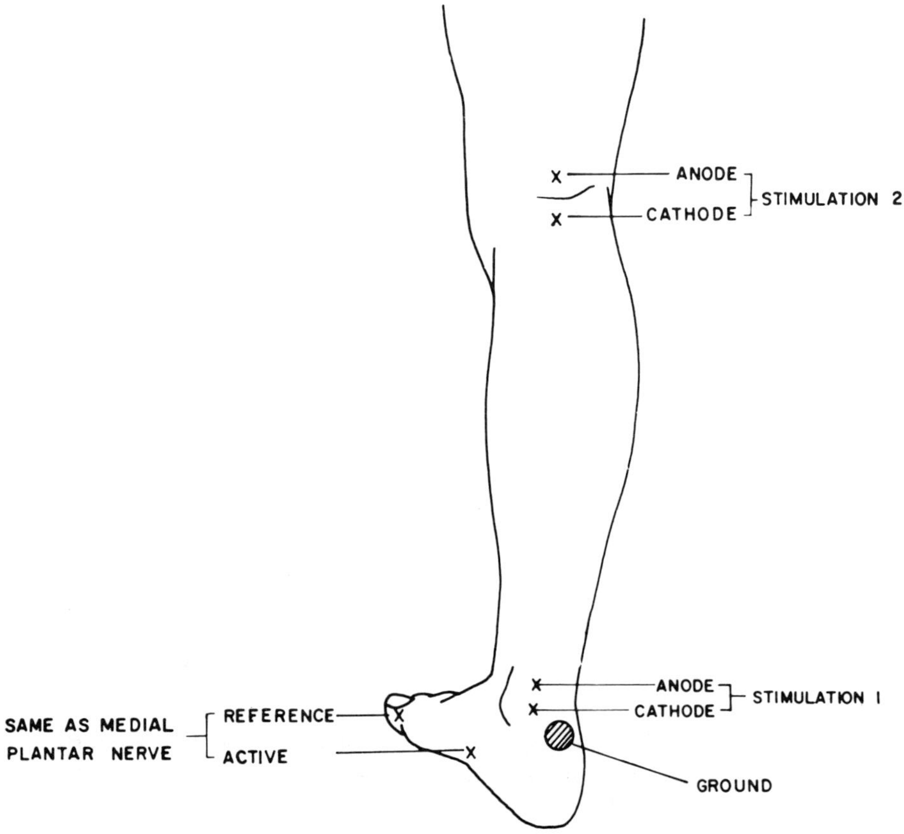

Figure 34 Tibial nerve motor nerve conduction velocity to the abductor hallucis muscle.

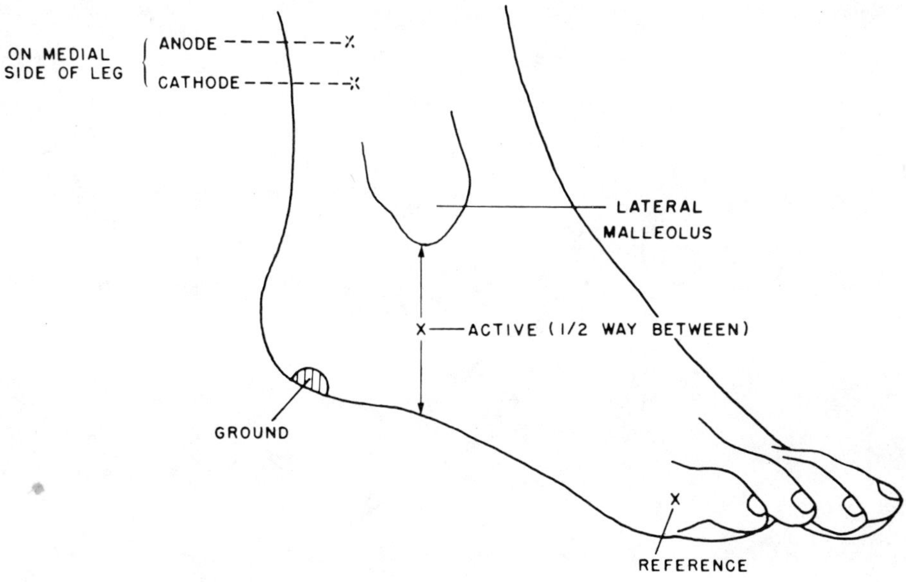

Figure 35 Lateral plantar nerve motor latency to the abductor digiti minimi muscle.

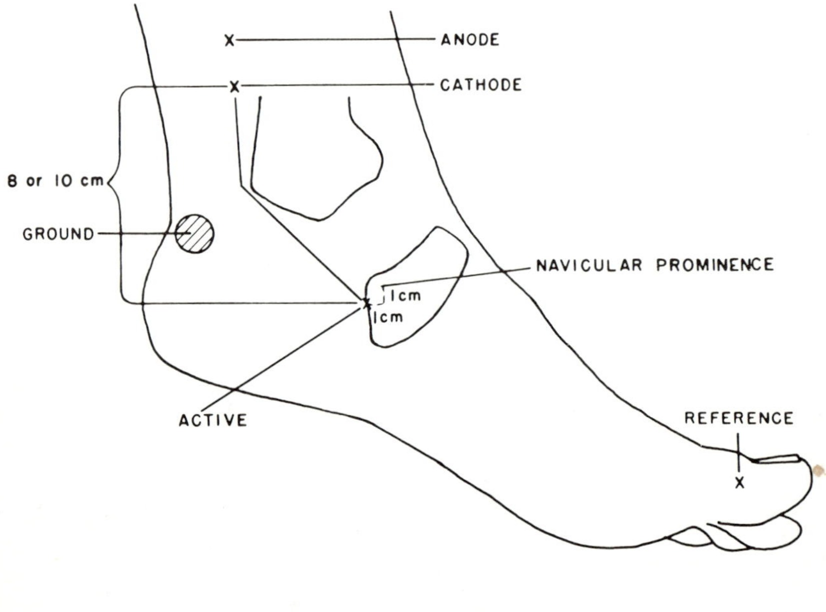

Figure 36 Medial plantar nerve motor latency to the abductor hallucis muscle.

Tibial Nerve Sensory Nerve Conduction Velocity (SNCV)—Medial Plantar and Lateral Plantar

Pickup: The active electrode is placed above the flexor retinaculum for both medial and lateral plantar nerves.

Ground: The ground is placed on the dorsum of the foot.

Stimulation:

Orthodromically:

Medial plantar—Stimulation is applied by means of a ring electrode on the great toe.

Lateral plantar—Stimulation is applied by means of a ring electrode on the fifth toe.

Electromyograph settings:

- Frequency—8 Hz or 1.6 kHz
- Sweep speed—2 or 5 msec/div
- Gain—5 to 10 μV

Distance: For the medial plantar nerve, the distance is measured with a tape from the first digit ring electrode to the ankle pickup. For the lateral plantar nerve, calipers are used to measure the distance from the fifth digit ring electrode to the ankle pickup. No specific standard distance was noted.

Oh SJ, Sarala PK, Kuba T, Elmore RS: Tarsal tunnel syndrome: Electrophysiological study. *Ann Neurol* 5:327–330, 1979.

Normal values: (*N* = 20 adults)

	Terminal SNCV	Mean amplitude
Medial plantar	35.22 ± 3.63 m/sec (mean ± 1 SD)	3.61 μV (range 2 to 6)
Lateral plantar	31.68 ± 4.39 m/sec (mean ± 1 SD)	1.89 μV (range 1 to 5)

Interval from the stimulus artifact to the negative peak of the compound sensory nerve action potential.

Comments: An averager must be used (the averager used 32 to 256 stimulations). Skin temperature was taken on the sole of the foot and measured 29.5 to 33.5°C.

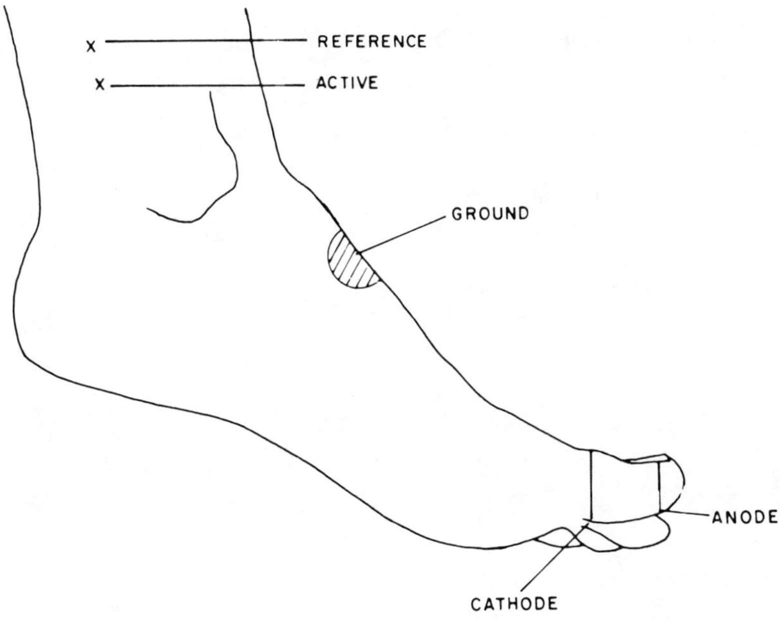

Figure 37 Medial plantar sensory nerve conduction velocity (orthodromic technique).

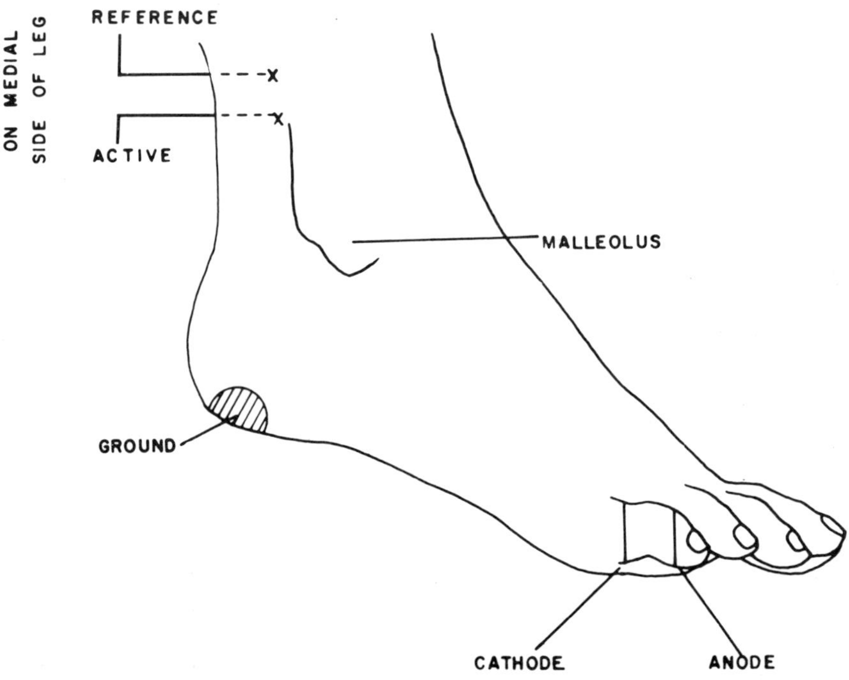

Figure 38 Lateral plantar sensory nerve conduction velocity (orthodromic technique).

H-Wave Latency

Pickup: The patient is prone with the feet suspended over the edge of the table or with a pillow placed under the ankles. The active surface electrode is placed on a point of bisection on the line connecting the popliteal crease and the proximal flare of the medial malleolus.

Reference: The reference is placed over the Achilles tendon.

Ground: The ground is placed between the sites of stimulation and pickup. This is especially important in H reflexes and minimizes artifacts.

Stimulation: Low-intensity current (*submaximal stimulus*) is used. The *cathode is proximal* (reverse of normal) and is placed over the tibial nerve in the popliteal fossa at the level of the popliteal crease. The nerve is just lateral to the popliteal artery or at the midpopliteal crease. (Note: a common error is to stimulate the peroneal nerve, which gives a wave that can be mistaken for the H reflex. Check for gastrocnemius contraction and the absence of peroneal contraction.)

Distance: Leg length is measured from the site of stimulation in the midpopliteal crease to the medial malleolus. (Note: this is not the tip of the medial malleolus, but represents a point over the tibial nerve just before it passes behind the most proximal part of the medial malleolus.)

Braddom RL, Johnson EW: Standardization of H reflex and diagnostic use in S1 radiculopathy. *Arch Phys Med Rehabil* 55:161–166, 1974.

Electromyograph settings:

- Frequency—8 Hz to 8 kHz
- Sweep speed—10 msec/div
- Gain—200 or 500 μV
- Intensity of stimulus—approximately 25 to 30 V
- Frequency of stimulus—0.5 pulses/sec
- Duration of the stimulus—1.0 msec

Normal values: ($N = 100$)

$$\text{Predicted H latency (msec)} = 9.14 + 0.46 \times \text{leg length (cm)} + 0.1 \times \text{age (years)}$$

$$2\ \text{SD} = 5.5\ \text{msec}$$

A difference between two legs of 1.2 msec (3 SEs) may be considered significant, assuming equal leg lengths.

Comments:

1. The H wave is thought to be due to the H reflex, a monosynaptic reflex evoked by direct electrical stimulation of large group Ia afferent fibers.

2. The H wave is recognized as an unchanging muscle evoked action potential which occurs at a latency of 28 to 35 msec in normals when measured from the gastrocnemius-soleus muscle in adults. It appears at *submaximal* stimulus, either before or shortly after the appearance of the M response. With increase in stimulus intensity the maximal H wave can be seen when the M response is submaximal. Further increases in the stimulus intensity increase the amplitude of the M response and reduce the amplitude of the H wave. At supramaximal stimulus, the H wave disappears and is sometimes replaced by an F wave.

3. Dr. Johnson suggests measuring latency and comparing it to predicted value. If latency is prolonged, or history and physical are highly suggestive of radiculopathy, then contralateral latency should be determined. A 1.2 msec or greater difference may be significant. In addition, an abnormal H reflex latency requires evaluation of sensory conduction (e.g., sural nerve) and motor conduction (e.g., tibial or peroneal nerve) to rule out neuropathy.

4. The H wave is normally present at birth, but after the age of 6 months it is present only in the gastrocnemius-soleus muscle, and can occasionally be recorded from the hamstrings and quadriceps muscles.

5. The H wave is triphasic with an initial positive deflection and a large negative deflection in the gastrocnemius-soleus muscle.

6. Active contraction of the antagonist muscle can inhibit the H reflex.

7. Marked shortening or lengthening of the muscle from which the H wave is being recorded can inhibit the reflex.

8. Sleep may also inhibit the reflex.

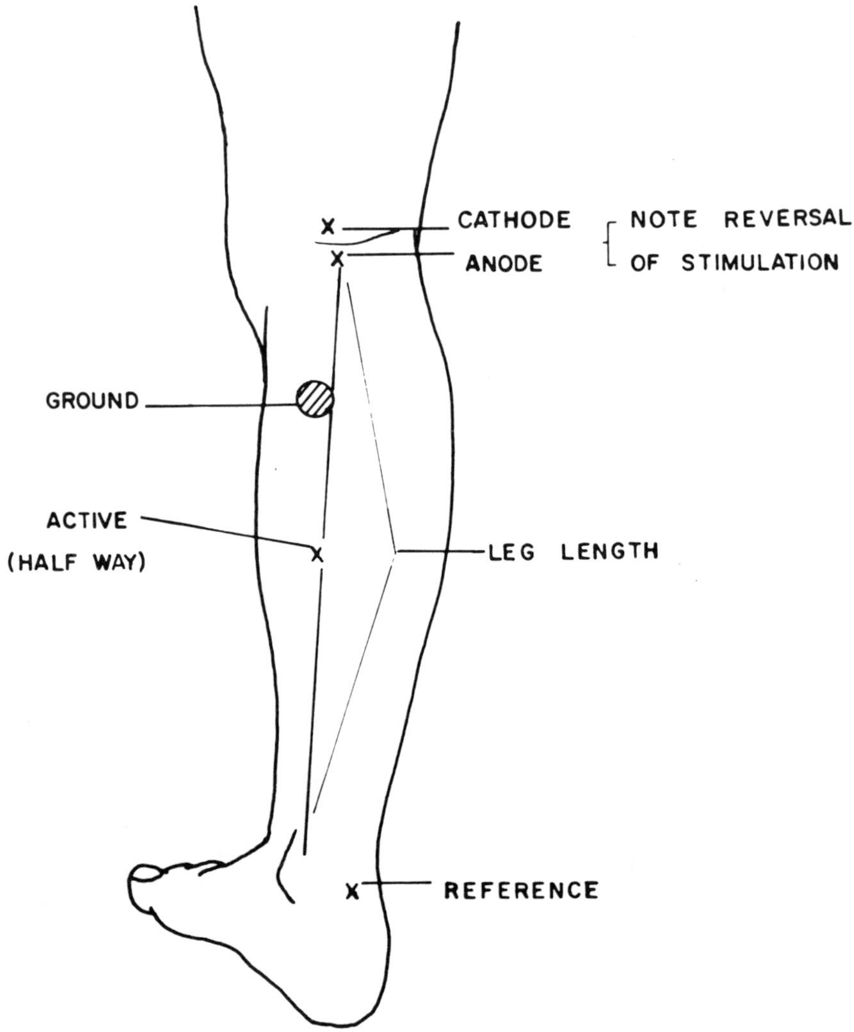

Figure 39 H-wave latency.

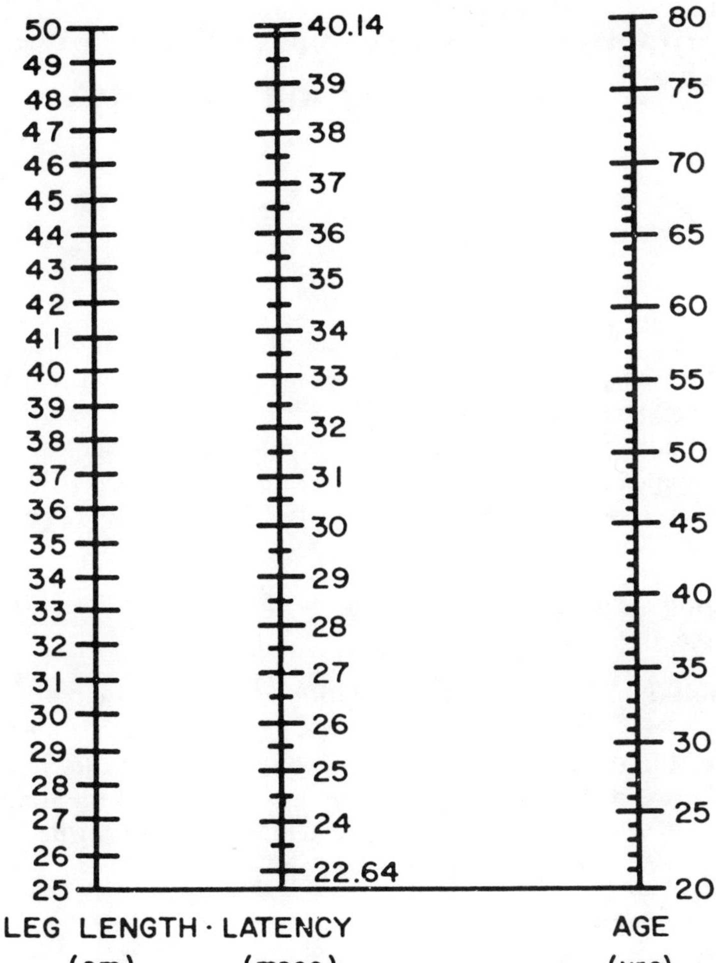

Figure 40 Nomogram of the simultaneous regression of H-wave latency on leg length and age. (From Braddom, Johnson: *Arch Phys Med Rehabil* 51:164–169, 1970, with permission.)

Saphenous Sensory Nerve Latency and Nerve Conduction Velocity

Pickup: The distal (reference) electrode is placed anterior to the highest prominence of the medial malleolus of the tibia, in the space between the malleolus and the medial border of the tibialis anterior tendon. The proximal active electrode is located 3 cm above the reference and just medial to the aforementioned tendon, whose direction is parallel to a line drawn between recording electrodes.

Ground: The ground is placed between the stimulation and pickup sites.

Stimulation: **Antidromic** stimulation is applied 14 cm above the proximal recording electrode and deep to the medial border of the tibia. Firm pressure is exerted, pushing the electrodes between the medial gastrocnemius muscle and the tibia. The cathode is distal. The gastrocnemius muscle can be relaxed by positioning it in plantarflexion.

Electromyograph settings:

- Frequency—8 Hz to 1.6 kHz
- Sweep speed—5 msec/div
- Gain—10 μV

Wainapel SF, Kim DJ, Ebel A: Conduction studies of the saphenous nerve in healthy subjects. *Arch Phys Med Rehabil* 59:316–319, 1978.

Normal values: ($N = 40$ adults)

$$\text{Velocity} = \frac{\text{sensory latency}}{\text{interelectrode distance}}$$

$$= 41.7 \pm 3.4 \text{ m/sec (mean} \pm 1 \text{ SD)}$$

Latency to negative peak of the evoked compound sensory nerve action potential—3.6 ± 0.4 msec (mean ± 1 SD); amplitude—9.0 ± 3.4 μV (mean ± 1 SD).

Comments: The main problem is that the gain is often 5 μV or less, which requires averaging. Since the sural nerve gives higher amplitudes, it is often the preferred nerve to study. Room temperature was maintained at 22.8°C during the study. The limbs were covered during the procedure.

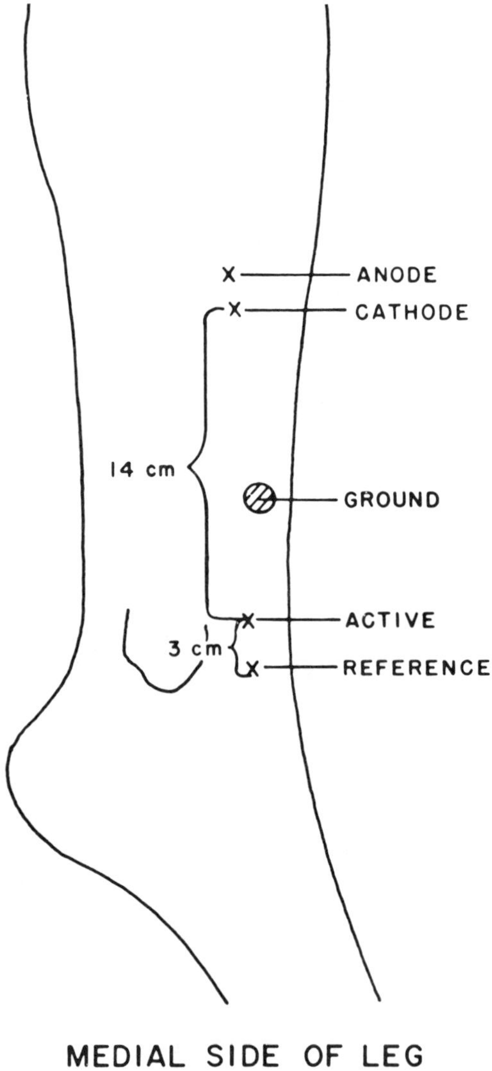

Figure 41 Saphenous nerve latency and nerve conduction velocity (antidromic technique).

Sural Sensory Nerve Latency

Pickup: The active is posterior and below the distal lateral malleolus of the fibula.

Reference: The reference is placed 3 cm distally.

Ground: The ground is placed between the cathode and the active pickup.

Stimulation: Stimulation is applied slightly lateral to the midline in the lower third of the posterior aspect of the leg with the cathode distally. The patient feels shocks radiate to the heel and foot. Sites 10, 14, or 17 cm from the active electrode are stimulated antidromically.

Electromyograph settings:

- Frequency—8 Hz to 1.6 kHz
- Sweep speed—5 msec/div
- Gain—10 μV

Schuchmann JA: Sural nerve conduction: A standardized technique. *Arch Phys Med Rehabil* 58:166–168, 1977.

Normal values:

Latency to peak:

Distance measured	Mean latency
10 cm	2.84 ± 0.27 msec (mean ± 1 SD; N = 37); range—2.3 to 3.38 msec
14 cm	3.50 ± 0.25 msec (mean ± 1 SD; N = 56); range—3.0 to 4.0 msec
17 cm	4.02 ± 0.30 msec (mean ± 1 SD; N = 56); range—3.42 to 4.62 msec
20 cm	4.58 ± 0.36 msec (mean ± 1 SD; N = 54); range—3.86 to 5.3 msec

Amplitude of evoked sensory potential—5 to 30 μV.

Comments: Tests at 14 and 17 cm were most easily evoked. An averager was not necessary. Limb temperatures were not recorded, but any limbs that were cool to palpation were warmed or excluded from the study.

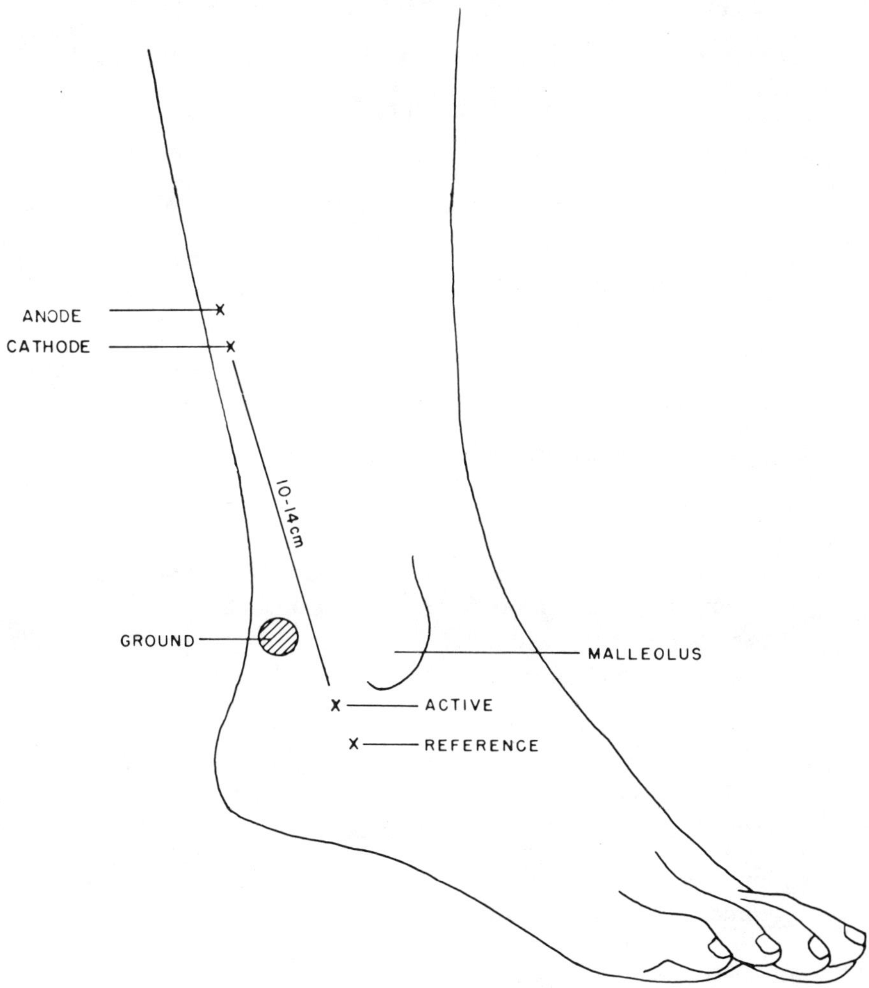

Figure 42 Sural sensory nerve latency (antidromic technique).

Motor Nerve Conduction Velocity Studies in Premature Infants, Infants, and Children

1. The motor nerve conduction velocity (MNCV) values of newborn are about half those of adults.

2. By age 3, the MNCV values are in the lower adult range.

3. By the age of 5, the MNCV values are essentially the same as those for adults.

4. Premature infant values (Cerra and Johnson)
   a. Premature ulnar MNCV ($N = 19$)—20.2 ± 2.6 m/sec (mean ± 1 SD); range—16.5 to 24.6 m/sec.
   b. Premature peroneal MNCV ($N = 17$)—19.1 ± 4.2 m/sec (mean ± 1 SD); range—13.7 to 28.3 m/sec.

5. The MNCV for the median, peroneal, and ulnar nerves for term infants, children, and adolescents are graphed in Figs. 43, 44, and 45. These figures, which express the mean ± 2 SD, are derived from the work of Ingrid Gamstorp.

6. In children, the medial and posterior tibial nerves are the most readily accessible for study.

Cerra D, Johnson EW: Motor conduction velocity in premature infants. *Arch Phys Med Rehabil* 43:160–164, 1962.

Gamstorp I: Normal conduction velocity of ulnar, median and peroneal nerves in infancy, childhood and adolescence. *Acta Paediatr Scand* **[Suppl]** 146:68–76, 1963.

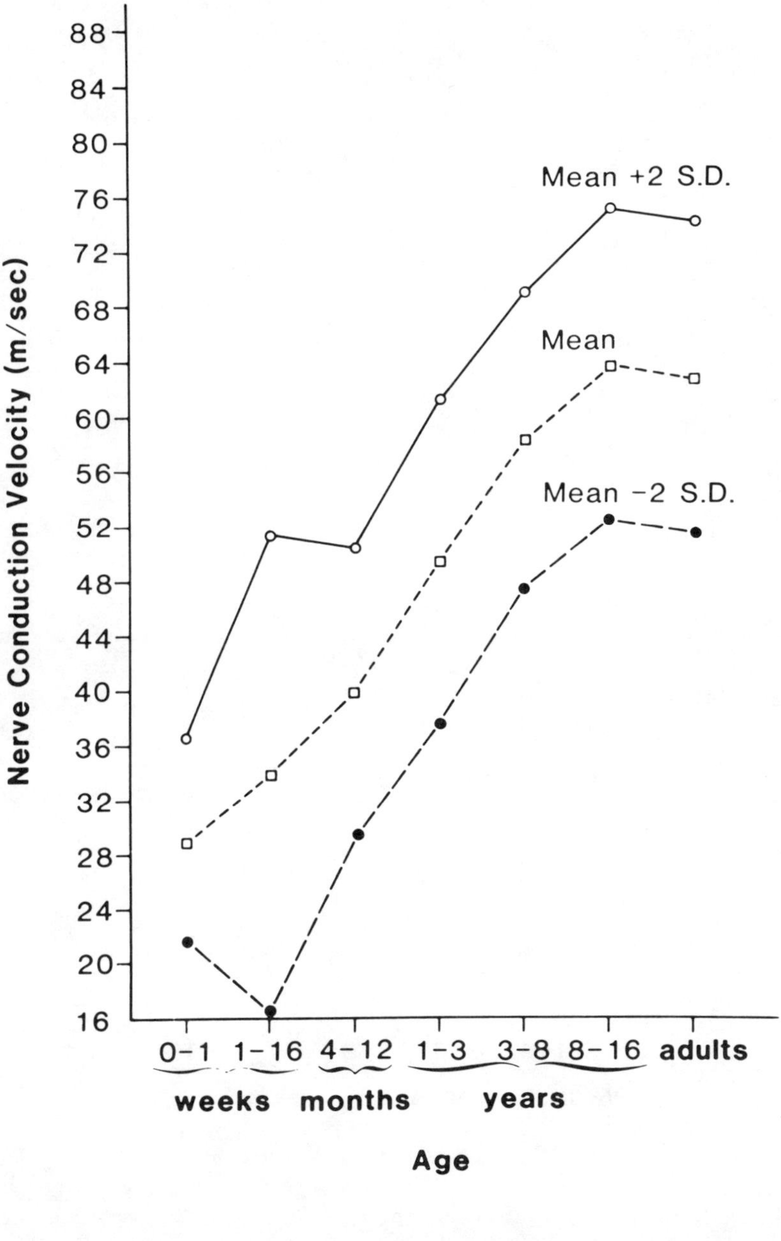

Figure 43 Median motor nerve conduction velocity (mean ± 2 SD) for term infants, children, and adolescents.

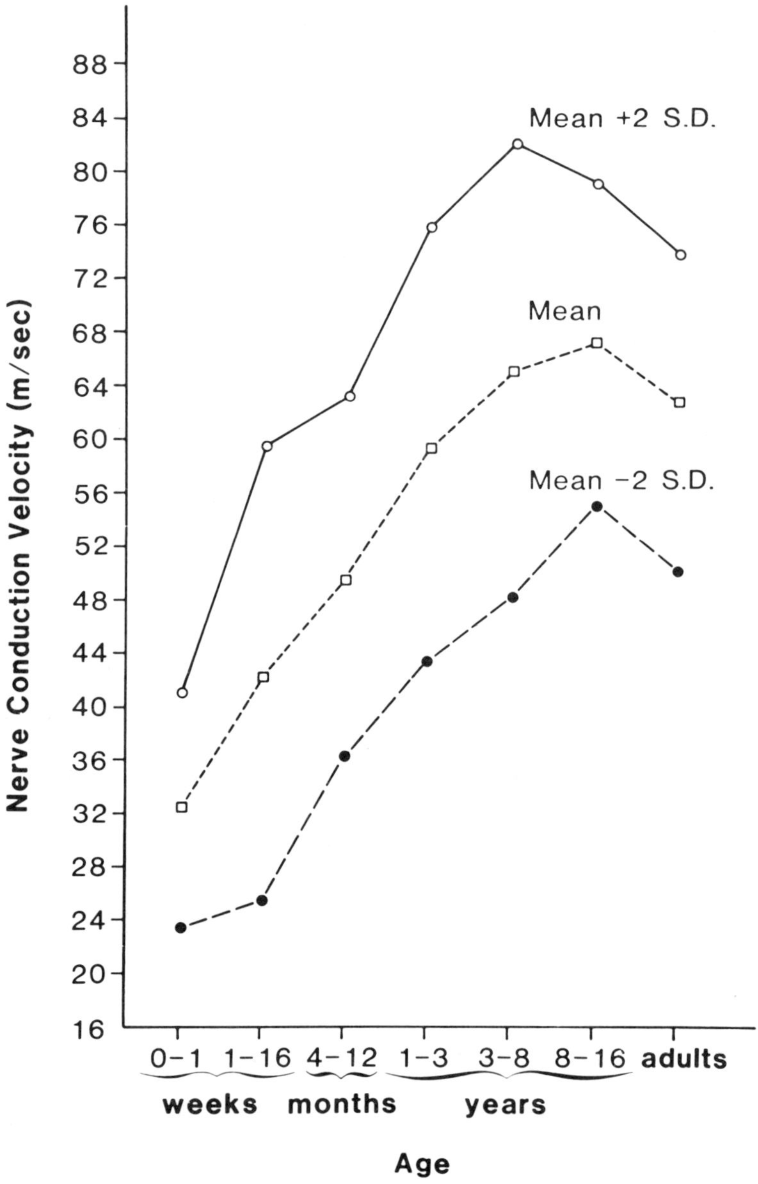

Figure 44 Ulnar motor nerve conduction velocity (mean ± 2 SD) for term infants, children, and adolescents.

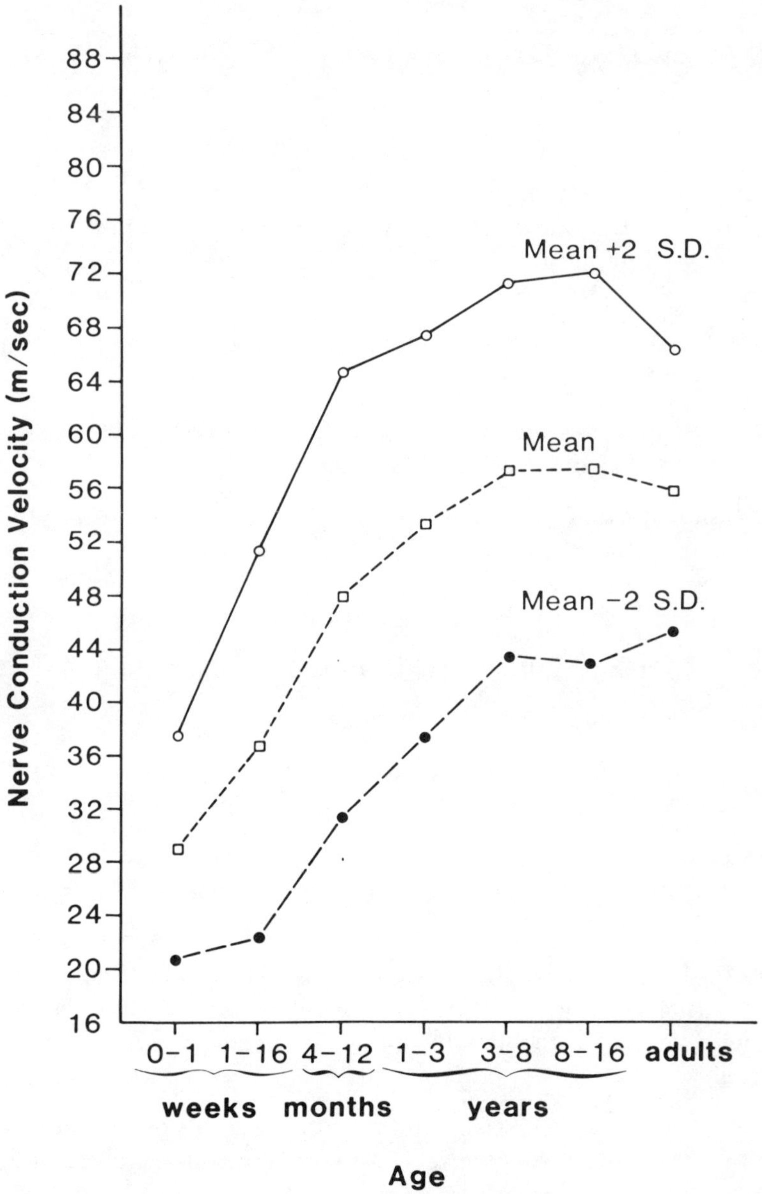

Figure 45 Peroneal motor nerve conduction velocity (mean ± 2 SD) for term infants, children, and adolescents.

Repetitive Stimulation (NM Junction)

Repetitive stimulation techniques can be useful in diagnosing diseases of the neuromuscular junction. However, technical errors can give erroneous results, and careful attention to technique is essential.

1. For 24 hr prior to testing, the patient must receive no medication that affects the neuromuscular junction.

2. The results must be printed on light-sensitive paper or stored and photographed for accurate measurement.

3. The muscle and joint(s) it crosses are immobilized to minimize movement artifact, and the stimulating and recording electrodes are secured to avoid any movement. Immobilization is best with the muscles stretched and joint(s) extended.

4. The skin temperature is 34°C (94°F) to avoid false negatives.

5. All stimuli must be *supramaximal.*

6. In myasthenic syndrome (Eaton-Lambert syndrome), the deficit is present in any muscle tested.

7. If the patient is suspected of having botulism, any clinically weak muscle is tested.

8. In myasthenia gravis muscle weakness increases with exertion but improves with rest and with anticholinesterase drugs. Proximal muscle testing is much more sensitive than distal. However, testing proximal is technically more difficult.

Proximal stimulation:

a. *Facial nerve:* **Stimulate** at the angle of the jaw with the **active** electrode over the nasalis muscle. Use a 2 × 2 to act as a compression dressing filling the void at the side of the nose.

b. *Upper trunk brachial plexus*: **Stimulate** at Erb's point with the **active** electrode over the deltoid muscle. This technique is painful and movement artifact can be a problem.

c. *Musculocutaneous nerve*: **Stimulate** in the axilla with the **active** electrode over the biceps brachii muscle. With this technique the stimulus can be unstable.

d. *Femoral nerve*: **Stimulate** in the inguinal region with the **active** electrode over the vastus medialis muscle. This technique can be painful.

Distal stimulation:

a. *Ulnar nerve*: Most investigators test the ulnar nerve distally. **Stimulate** the ulnar nerve at the wrist with the **active** electrode over the abductor digiti minimi muscle.

b. *Median nerve*: **Stimulate** the median nerve at the wrist with the **active** electrode over the abductor pollicis brevis muscle. The disadvantage of this technique is that the thumb is hard to immobilize.

9. During each portion of the test (the single response, the 2/sec stimulation, the 10 sec post-exercise), the potential amplitude often decreases during the first four responses. Thus most investigators measure the fifth response, compare its amplitude to that of the first response of the train, and calculate the percentage of change.

10. In a rigidly controlled system, a decrement by the fifth successive potential (as compared to the first) of 10% is definitely abnormal in distal muscles. In proximal muscles, where rigid control is more difficult to obtain, only decrements of over 20% are considered abnormal.

11. The following are important to observe during testing:
  a. Amplitude of the initial response to a single nerve supramaximal stimulation.
  b. Presence or absence of a decrement during repetitive stimulation at a slow rate.

c. Presence or absence of a decrement or increment after isometric exercise and then stimulation at a slow rate.
d. Postactivation facilitation.
e. Postactivation exhaustion.
f. Change in response after anticholinesterase drugs.

12. **Actual technique:**
    a. To obtain the single response: in an unexercised muscle initially use a high voltage to obtain a supramaximal response, then look at the peak-to-peak amplitude of the initial muscle action potential.
    b. Wait 1 min before stimulating at a frequency of 2 or 3/sec for 3 sec, looking for a decrement. For screening purposes, a train of 3 to 5 stimuli is adequate. To test reproducibility of the decrement, a muscle must be rested 1 min between tests.
    c. Wait at least 1 min (until the amplitude is back to the initial amplitude and use it as the baseline before exercise) before having the patient perform isometric exercises for 10 sec (30 sec if the muscle is not clinically weak).
    d. Ten seconds after the exercise facilitation is completed, start to stimulate at 2 or 3/sec for 3 sec. Repeat this at 30 sec and at 1, 2, 3, and 5 min to check for *postactivation exhaustion or facilitation.* (According to the literature, 2 min appears to be the most sensitive time.)

13. Figure 46 indicates results seen with repetitive stimulation in normals and in patients with myasthenia gravis, myasthenic syndrome, and botulism.

14. A more sensitive method to evaluate the status of the neuromuscular junction is Jitter study of a motor fiber pair by single-fiber electromyography.

15. Each laboratory should establish its approach and technique to evaluate possible dysfunction of the neuromuscular junction. Technique is perfected by performing a number of tests on normal subjects.

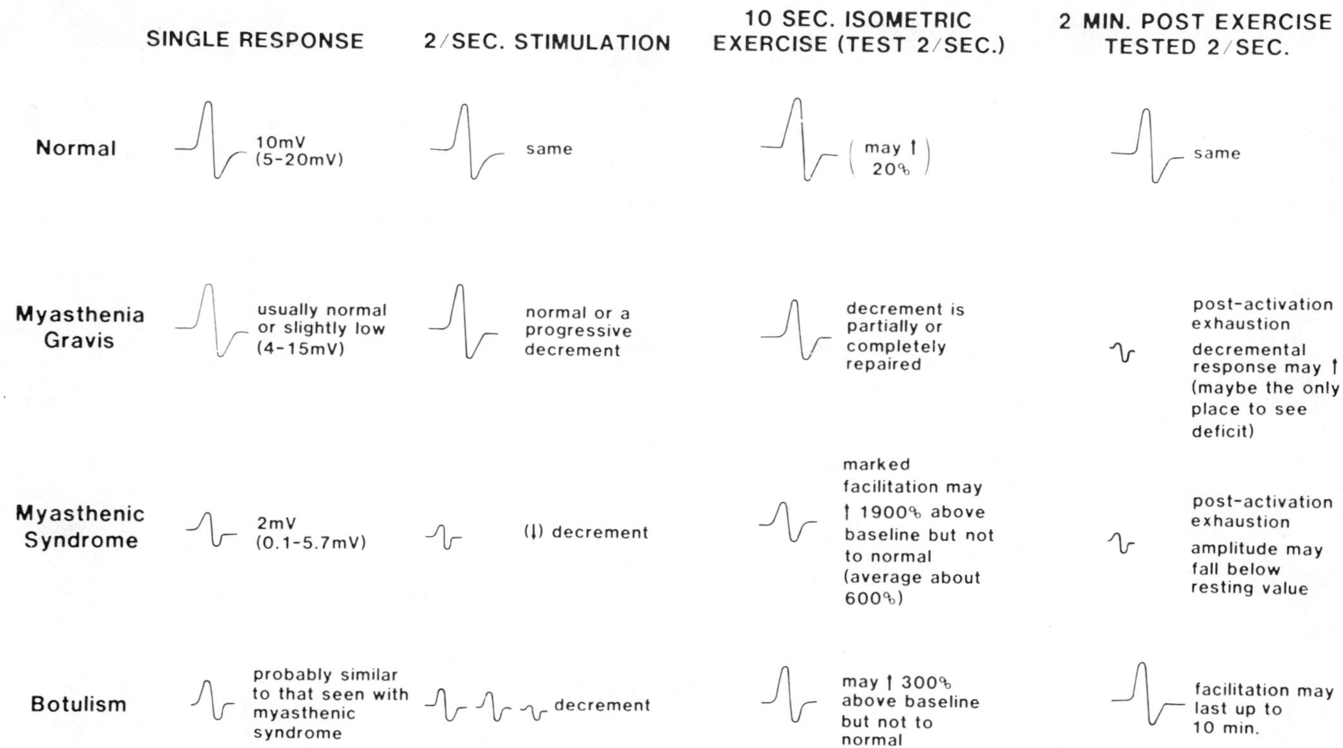

Figure 46 Repetitive stimulation (a decrement must be reproducible on a number of trials).

Glossary of Terms Used in Clinical Electromyography

Compiled by the Nomenclature Committee, American Association of Electromyography and Electrodiagnosis*

ABSOLUTE REFRACTORY PERIOD See *Refractory Period.*

ACCOMMODATION The reduced efficacy of a prolonged constant current or a gradually increasing current in generating action potentials from nervous tissue.

ACCOMMODATION CURVE A curve obtained by plotting the strength of current (in multiples of *Rheobase*) required to produce a response from an excitable tissue against the time required by a slowly rising current pulse to reach that value.

ACTION CURRENT The electrical current associated with an *Action Potential.*

ACTION POTENTIAL (Abbr. *AP*). Strictly defined, the all-or-none, self-propagating, nondecrementing voltage change recorded from an excitable cell. The source of the action potential should be specified, e.g., nerve (fiber) action potential or muscle (fiber) action potential. Commonly, the term refers to the nearly synchronous summated action potentials of a group of cells, e.g., *Motor Unit Potential.* To avoid ambiguity in reference to the recording of nearly synchronous summated action potentials of nerve and muscle as done in nerve conduction studies, it is recommended that the terms *Compound Nerve Action Potential* and *Compound Muscle Action Potential* be used, respectively, or the specific named responses, e.g., *M Wave, F Wave, H Wave, R1 and R2 Waves.*

---

* George H. Kraft, *Chairman;* Jasper R. Daube, Joel A. DeLisa, Joseph Goodgold, Charles K. Jablecki, Edward H. Lambert, J. A. Simpson, Albrecht Struppler, David O. Wiechers. Reprinted with permission of the American Association of Electromyography and Electrodiagnosis.

ACTIVE ELECTRODE Synonymous with *Exploring Electrode.* See *Recording Electrode.*

ADAPTATION A transient state at the initiation of an abrupt depolarization in which the impulse frequency first increases and then diminishes before the cell reaches a steady firing frequency.

AFTER DISCHARGE Repetitive electrical firing that persists after initiation by some other process, usually muscle contraction. It may have variable form and be regular or irregular at long or short intervals.

AFTERPOTENTIAL Membrane potential following the spike component of an *Action Potential* and not yet returned to a steady resting value. It first has a positive phase (positive afterpotential), which is followed by a negative phase (negative afterpotential).

AMPLITUDE With reference to an *Action Potential,* the maximum voltage difference between two points, usually baseline to peak or peak to peak. By convention, the amplitude of the *Compound Muscle Action Potential* is measured from the baseline to the most negative peak. In contrast, the amplitude of a *Compound Sensory Nerve Action Potential, Motor Unit Potential, Fibrillation Potential, Positive Sharp Wave, Fasciculation Potential,* and most other *Action Potentials* is measured from the most positive to the most negative peak.

ANODAL BLOCK A local block of nerve conduction caused by hyperpolarization of the nerve cell membrane by an electrical stimulus. See *Stimulating Electrode.*

ANODE The positive terminal of a source of electrical current.

ANTIDROMIC Said of an action potential or of the stimulation causing the action potential that propagates in the direction opposite to the normal (dromic or *Orthodromic*) one for that fiber—i.e., conduction along motor fibers toward the spinal cord and conduction along sensory fibers away from the spinal cord. Contrast with *Orthodromic.*

ARTIFACT A voltage change generated by a biological or nonbiological source other than the ones of interest. The *Stimulus Artifact* is the potential recorded at the time the stimulus is applied and includes the *Electrical* or *Shock Artifact,* which is a potential due to the volume conducted electrical stimulus. The stimulus and shock artifacts usually precede the activity of interest. A *Movement Artifact* refers to a change in the recorded activity due to movement of the recording electrodes.

AUDITORY EVOKED POTENTIAL Electrical waveform of biological origin elicited by a sound stimulus. See *Evoked Potential.*

BACKFIRING Recurrent discharge of an antidromically activated motor neuron.

BAER Abbreviation for brain stem auditory evoked response. Synonym: *Brain Stem Auditory Evoked Potential.*

BASELINE The potential difference recorded from the biological system of interest while the system is at rest.

BENIGN FASCICULATION Use of term discouraged. See *Fasciculation Potential.*

BER Abbreviation for brain stem evoked response. See *Brain Stem Auditory Evoked Potential.*

BIFILAR NEEDLE ELECTRODE See *Bipolar Needle Electrode.*

BIPHASIC ACTION POTENTIAL An action potential with two phases.

BIPHASIC SPIKE POTENTIAL See *End-Plate Activity, Biphasic.*

BIPOLAR NEEDLE ELECTRODE A recording electrode with two insulated wires side by side in a metal cannula whose bare tips act as the active and reference electrodes. The metal cannula may be grounded.

BIZARRE HIGH-FREQUENCY DISCHARGE See *Complex Repetitive Discharge.*

BIZARRE REPETITIVE POTENTIAL See *Complex Repetitive Discharge.*

BLINK REFLEX See *Blink Responses.*

BLINK RESPONSE Strictly defined, one of the *Blink Responses.* See *Blink Responses.*

BLINK RESPONSES *Compound Muscle Action Potentials* evoked from orbicularis oculi muscles as a result of brief electrical or mechanical stimuli to the cutaneous area innervated by the supraorbital (or less commonly the infraorbital) branch of the trigeminal nerve. Typically, there is an early compound muscle action potential (*R1 Wave*) ipsilateral to the stimulation site with a latency of about 10 msec and a bilateral late compound muscle action potential (*R2 Wave*) with a latency of approximately 30 msec. Generally, only the *R2 Wave* is associated with a visible twitch of the orbicularis oculi. The configuration, amplitude, duration, and latency of the two components, along with the sites of recording and the sites of stimulation, should be specified. Both *R1* and *R2 Waves* are probably due to a polysynaptic brain stem reflex, the *Blink Reflex,* with the afferent arc provided by the sensory branches of the trigeminal nerve and the efferent arc provided by the facial nerve motor fibers.

BRAIN STEM AUDITORY EVOKED POTENTIAL (Abbr. *BAEP*). Early (latency less than 10 msec) electrical waveforms of biological origin elicited in response to sound stimuli. See *Evoked Potential.*

BRAIN STEM AUDITORY EVOKED RESPONSE (Abbr. *BAER, BER*). Synonymous with *Brain Stem Auditory Evoked Potential.*

BREAKTHROUGH VOLUNTARY ACTIVITY A burst of voluntary activity occurring within the *S-X Interval.*

BSAP Abbreviation for brief, small, abundant potentials. Use of term is discouraged. It is used to describe a recruitment pattern of brief-duration, small-amplitude, overly abundant motor unit action potentials. Quantitative measurements of motor unit potential duration, amplitude, numbers of phases, and recruitment frequency are to be preferred to qualitative descriptions such as this. See *Motor Unit Potential.*

BSAPP Abbreviation for brief, small, abundant, polyphasic potentials. Use of term is discouraged. It is used to describe a recruitment pattern of brief-duration, small-amplitude, overly abundant, polyphasic motor unit action potentials. Quantitative measurements of motor unit potential duration, amplitude, numbers of phases, and recruitment frequency are to be preferred to qualitative descriptions such as this. See *Motor Unit Potential.*

CATHODE The negative terminal of a source of electrical current.

CEREBRAL EVOKED POTENTIAL Electrical waveforms of biological origin recorded over the head and elicited by sensory stimuli. See specific evoked potentials, e.g., *Somatosensory Evoked Potential, Visual Evoked Potential, Auditory Evoked Potential.*

CHRONAXIE The time required for an electrical current stimulus at a voltage twice the *Rheobase* to elicit the first visible muscle twitch. See *Strength-Duration Curve.*

CLINICAL ELECTROMYOGRAPHY Loosely used to refer to all electrodiagnostic studies of peripheral nerves and muscle. See *Electrodiagnosis.*

COAXIAL NEEDLE ELECTRODE See synonym, *Concentric Needle Electrode.*

COLLISION When used with reference to nerve conduction studies, the interaction of two action potentials propagated toward each other from opposite directions on the same nerve fiber so that the refractory periods of the two potentials prevent propagation past each other.

COMPLEX ACTION POTENTIAL See preferred term, *Serrated Action Potential.*

COMPLEX MOTOR UNIT POTENTIAL See preferred term, *Serrated Action Potential.*

COMPLEX REPETITIVE DISCHARGE Polyphasic or serrated action potentials that may begin spontaneously or after a needle movement. They have a uniform frequency, shape, and amplitude, with abrupt onset, cessation, or change in configuration. Amplitude ranges from 100 μV to 1 mV and frequency of discharge from 5 to 100 Hz.

COMPOUND ACTION POTENTIAL See *Compound Mixed Nerve Action Potential, Compound Motor Nerve Action Potential, Compound*

Nerve Action Potential, Compound Sensory Nerve Action Potential, and Compound Muscle Action Potential.

COMPOUND MIXED NERVE ACTION POTENTIAL A compound nerve action potential is considered to have been evoked from afferent and efferent fibers if the recording electrodes detect activity on a mixed nerve with the electrical stimulus applied to a segment of the nerve which contains both afferent and efferent fibers.

COMPOUND MOTOR NERVE ACTION POTENTIAL A compound nerve action potential is considered to have been evoked from efferent fibers to a muscle if the recording electrodes detect activity only in a motor nerve or a motor branch of a mixed nerve, or if the electrical stimulus is applied only to such a nerve or a ventral root. The amplitude, latency, duration, and phases should be noted. See *Compound Nerve Action Potential.*

COMPOUND MUSCLE ACTION POTENTIAL The summation of nearly synchronous muscle fiber action potentials recorded from a muscle commonly produced by stimulation of the nerve supplying the muscle either directly or indirectly. Baseline-to-peak amplitude, duration, and latency of the negative phase should be noted, along with details of the method of stimulation and recording. Use of specific named potentials is recommended, e.g., *M Wave, F Wave, H Wave,* and *R1 Wave* or *R2 Wave* (*Blink Responses*).

COMPOUND NERVE ACTION POTENTIAL The summation of nearly synchronous nerve fiber action potentials recorded from a nerve trunk, commonly produced by stimulation of the nerve directly or indirectly. Details of the method of stimulation and recording should be specified, together with the fiber type (sensory, motor, or mixed).

COMPOUND SENSORY NERVE ACTION POTENTIAL A compound nerve action potential is considered to have been evoked from afferent fibers if the recording electrodes detect activity only in a sensory nerve or in a sensory branch of a mixed nerve, or if the electrical stimulus is applied to such a nerve or a dorsal nerve root, or an adequate stimulus is applied synchronously to sensory receptors. The amplitude, latency, duration, and configuration should be noted. Generally, the amplitude is measured as the maximum peak-to-peak voltage, the latency as either the *Latency* to the initial deflection or the *Peak Latency* to the negative peak, and the duration as the interval from the first deflection of the waveform from the baseline to its final return to the baseline. The compound sensory nerve action potential has been referred to as the *Sensory Response* or *Sensory Potential.*

CONCENTRIC NEEDLE ELECTRODE Recording electrode that measures the potential difference between the bare tip of a central insulated wire in the bare shaft of a metal cannula. The bare tip of the central wire (active electrode) is flush with the bevel of the cannula (reference electrode).

CONDITIONING STIMULUS A stimulus, preceding a *Test Stimulus,* used to modify the response elicited by the test stimulus alone. *See Stimulus.*

CONDUCTION BLOCK Failure of an action potential to be conducted past a particular point in the nervous system. In practice, a conduction block is documented by demonstration of a reduction in amplitude of an evoked potential greater than that normally seen with electrical stimulation at two different points on a nerve trunk; anatomical nerve variations and technical factors related to nerve stimulation must be excluded as the source of the reduction in amplitude.

CONDUCTION DISTANCE See *Conduction Velocity.*

CONDUCTION TIME See *Conduction Velocity.*

CONDUCTION VELOCITY Speed of propagation of an *Action Potential* along a nerve or muscle fiber. The nerve fiber studied (motor, sensory, autonomic, or mixed) should be specified. For a nerve trunk, the maximum conduction velocity is calculated from the *Latency* of the evoked potential (muscle or nerve) at maximal or supramaximal intensity of stimulation at two different points. The distance between the two points (*Conduction Distance*) is divided by the difference between the corresponding latencies (*Conduction Time*). The calculated velocity represents the conduction velocity of the fastest fibers and is expressed as meters per second (m/sec). As commonly used, the term *Conduction Velocity* refers to the *Maximum*

Conduction Velocity. By specialized techniques, the conduction velocity of other fibers can be determined as well and should be specified, e.g., minimum conduction velocity.

CONTRACTION A voluntary or involuntary reversible muscle shortening that may or may not be accompanied by *Action Potentials* from muscle. This term is to be contrasted with the term *Contracture,* which refers to a condition of fixed muscle shortening.

CONTRACTURE An electrically silent, involuntary state of maintained muscle contraction, as seen in phosphorylase deficiency. The term is also used to refer to immobility of a joint due to other local processes.

CORTICAL EVOKED POTENTIAL See *Cerebral Evoked Potential.*

COUPLED DISCHARGE See preferred term, *Late Component.*

CRAMP DISCHARGE Repetitive firing of action potentials with the configuration of *Motor Unit Potentials* at a high frequency in a large area of muscle, associated with an involuntary, painful muscle contraction (cramp).

CYCLES PER SECOND Unit of frequency (abbr. *C/sec* or *CPS*). Preferred equivalent is *Hertz* (abbr. *Hz*).

DECREMENTING RESPONSE A progressive decline in the amplitude associated with a decrease in the area of the negative phase of the *M Wave* of successive responses to a series of supramaximal stimuli. The rate of stimulation and the number of stimuli should be specified. Contrast with *Incrementing Response.*

DELAY Interval between onset of oscilloscope sweep and onset of a stimulus. Had been used in the past to designate the interval from the stimulus to the response. Compare with *Latency.*

DENERVATION POTENTIAL Use of term discouraged. See *Fibrillation Potential.*

DEPOLARIZATION A decrease in the electrical potential difference across a membrane from any cause, to any degree, relative to the normal resting potential. See *Polarization.*

DEPOLARIZATION BLOCK Failure of an excitable cell to respond to a stimulus because of *Depolarization* of the cell membrane.

DISCHARGE Synonymous with *Action Potential.*

DISCHARGE FREQUENCY The rate of repetition of an *Action Potential.* When potentials occur in groups, the rate of recurrence of the group and the rate of repetition of the individual components in the groups should be specified. See *Firing Rate.*

DISCRETE ACTIVITY The pattern of electrical activity at full voluntary contraction of the muscle is reduced to the extent that each individual *Motor Unit Potential* can be identified. The firing frequency of each of these potentials should be specified together with the force of contraction.

DISTAL LATENCY See *Motor Latency* and *Sensory Latency.*

"DIVE BOMBER" POTENTIAL Use of term discouraged. See preferred term, *Myotonic Discharge.*

DOUBLE DISCHARGE Two action potentials of the same form and nearly the same amplitude, occurring consistently in the same relationship to one another at intervals of 2 to 20 msec. Contrast with *Paired Discharge.*

DOUBLET Synonymous with *Double Discharge.*

DURATION The time during which something exists or acts. (1) The duration of individual potential *Waveforms* is defined as the interval from the first deflection from the baseline to its final return to the baseline, unless otherwise specified. One common exception is the duration of the *M Wave,* which usually refers to the interval from the deflection of the first negative phase from the baseline to its return to the baseline. (2) The duration of a single electrical stimulus refers to the interval of the applied current or voltage. (3) The duration of recurring stimuli or action potentials refers to the interval from the beginning to the end of the series.

EARTHING ELECTRODE Synonymous with *Ground Electrode.*

ELECTRICAL ARTIFACT See *Artifact.*

ELECTRICAL SILENCE The absence of measurable electrical activity due to biological or nonbiological sources. The sensitivity, or signal-to-noise level, of the recording system should be specified.

ELECTRODE A device capable of conducting electricity. The material (metal, fabric), size, configuration (disc, ring, needle), and location (surface, intramuscular, intracranial) should be specified. Electrodes may be used to record an electrical potential difference (*Recording Electrodes*) or to apply an electrical current (*Stimulating Electrodes*). In both cases, two electrodes are always required. Depending on the relative size and location of the electrodes, however, the stimulating or recording condition may be referred to as "*Monopolar.*" See *Ground Electrode, Recording Electrode,* and *Stimulating Electrode.* Also see specific needle electrode configurations: *Monopolar, Concentric, Bipolar,* and *Multilead Needle Electrodes.*

ELECTRODIAGNOSIS (Abbr. *EDX*). General term used to refer to the recording of responses of nerves and muscle to electrical stimulation and the recording of insertional, spontaneous, and voluntary action potentials from muscle. It was originally used to refer to *Strength-Duration Curve* determinations and other early techniques.

ELECTROMYELOGRAPHY The recording and study of electrical activity from the spinal cord. The term is also used to refer to studies of electrical activity from the cauda equina.

ELECTROMYOGRAM The record obtained by *Electromyography.*

ELECTROMYOGRAPH An instrument for detecting and displaying *Action Potentials* from muscle and nerve.

ELECTROMYOGRAPHY (Abbr. *EMG*). Strictly defined, the recording and study of insertional, spontaneous, and voluntary electrical activity of muscle. It is commonly used to refer to nerve conduction studies as well. Compare with *Clinical Electromyography* and the more general term, *Electrodiagnosis.*

ELECTRONEUROGRAPHY The recording and study of the action potentials of peripheral nerves. See preferred term, *Nerve Conduction Studies,* and the more general term, *Electrodiagnosis.*

ELECTRONEUROMYOGRAPHY A newly fabricated word used to

refer to the combined studies of *Electromyography* and *Electroneurography.* See preferred terms, *Clinical Electromyography* and *Electrodiagnosis.*

ELECTROSPINOGRAM The record obtained by *Electromyelography.*

END-PLATE ACTIVITY Spontaneous electrical activity recorded with a needle electrode close to muscle end-plates. May be either of two forms:

1. **MONOPHASIC:** Low-amplitude (10 to 20 μV), short-duration (0.5 to 1 msec), monophasic (negative) potentials that occur in a dense, steady pattern and are restricted to a localized area of the muscle. Because of the multitude of different potentials occurring, the exact frequency, although appearing to be high, cannot be defined. These potentials are miniature end-plate potentials recorded extracellularly. This form of end-plate activity has been referred to as *End-Plate Noise* and is associated with a sound not unlike that of a seashell, which has been called a *Seashell Noise* or *Roar.*
2. **BIPHASIC:** Moderate-amplitude (100 to 300 μV), short-duration (2 to 4 msec), biphasic (negative-positive) spike potentials that occur irregularly in short bursts with a high frequency (50 to 100 Hz), restricted to a localized area within the muscle. These potentials are generated by muscle fibers excited by activity in nerve terminals. These potentials have been referred to as *Biphasic Spike Potentials, End-Plate Spikes,* and, incorrectly, "*Nerve*" *Potentials.*

END-PLATE NOISE See *End-Plate Activity, Monophasic.*

END-PLATE POTENTIAL Graded, nonpropagated potential recorded by microelectrodes from muscle fibers in the region of the neuromuscular junction.

END-PLATE SPIKE See *End-Plate Activity, Biphasic.*

END-PLATE ZONE The site of the neuromuscular junction, a localized area of the muscle fiber in which activity identified as end-plate activity may be recorded.

EVOKED ACTION POTENTIAL Action potential elicited by a stimulus.

EVOKED COMPOUND MUSCLE ACTION POTENTIAL The electrical activity of a muscle produced by stimulation of the nerves supplying the muscle. Baseline-to-peak amplitude of the negative phase, duration of the negative phase, and *Latency* should be measured, and details of the method of stimulation should be recorded. See specific named potentials: *M Wave, F Wave, H Wave, R1* and *R2 Waves,* and *Blink Responses.*

EVOKED POTENTIAL Electrical waveform elicited by and temporally related to a stimulus, most commonly an electrical stimulus delivered to a sensory receptor or nerve, or applied directly to a discrete area of the brain, spinal cord, or muscle. See *Auditory Evoked Potential, Brain Stem Auditory Evoked Potential, Spinal Evoked Potential, Somatosensory Evoked Potential, Visual Evoked Potential, Cerebral Evoked Potential, Compound Muscle Action Potential,* and *Compound Sensory Nerve Action Potential.*

EVOKED RESPONSE Tautology. Use of term discouraged. Suggested term is *Evoked Potential.*

EXCITABILITY Capacity to be activated by or react to a stimulus.

EXCITATORY POSTSYNAPTIC POTENTIAL (Abbr. *EPSP*). A local, graded depolarization of a neuron in response to activation by a nerve terminal at a synapse. Contrast with *Inhibitory Postsynaptic Potential.*

EXPLORING ELECTRODE Synonymous with *Active Electrode.* See *Recording Electrode.*

FACILITATION OF NEUROMUSCULAR TRANSMISSION An increase in the amplitude of an end-plate potential of a muscle fiber with stimulation of the axon in a variety of physiological and pharmacological settings. Use of the term is not recommended for description of the phenomenon recorded in repetitive stimulation studies.

FASCICULATION The random, spontaneous twitching of a group of muscle fibers which may be visible through the skin. The electrical activity associated with the spontaneous contraction is called the *Fasciculation Potential.* Compare with *Myokymia.*

FASCICULATION POTENTIAL The electrical potential associated with *Fasciculation* which has dimensions of a motor unit potential that occurs spontaneously as a single discharge. Most commonly these potentials occur sporadically and are termed "single fasciculation potentials." Occasionally, the potentials occur as a grouped discharge and are termed "grouped fasciculation potentials." The occurrence of large numbers of either simple or grouped fasciculations may produce a writhing, vermicular movement of the skin called *Myokymia.* Use of the terms *Benign Fasciculation* and *Malignant Fasciculation* is discouraged. Instead, the configuration of the potentials, peak-to-peak amplitude, duration, number of phases, and stability of configuration, in addition to frequency of occurrence, should be specified.

FATIGUE Reduction in the force of contraction of muscle fibers as a result of repeated use or electrical stimulation. More generally, it is a state of depressed responsiveness resulting from protracted activity and requiring appreciable recovery time.

FIBER DENSITY (1) Anatomically, fiber density is a measure of the number of muscle or nerve fibers per unit area. (2) In single-fiber EMG, the fiber density is the mean number of muscle fiber potentials under voluntary control encountered during a systematic search. See *Single Fiber Electromyography.*

FIBRILLATION The spontaneous contractions of individual muscle fibers which are ordinarily not visible through the skin. This term has been used loosely in electromyography for the preferred term, *Fibrillation Potential.*

FIBRILLATION POTENTIAL The electrical activity associated with fibrillating muscle fibers, reflecting the action potential of a single muscle fiber. The action potentials may occur spontaneously or after movement of the needle electrode. The potentials usually occur repetitively and regularly. Classically, the potentials are biphasic spikes of short duration (usually less than 5 msec) with an initial positive phase and a peak-to-peak amplitude of less than 1 mV. The firing rate has a wide range (1 to 50 Hz) and often decreases just before cessation of an individual discharge. A high-pitched regular sound is associated with the discharge of fibrillation potentials and has been described in the old literature as "rain on a tin roof." In addition to this classic form of fibrillation potentials, *Positive Sharp Waves* may also be recorded from fibrillating muscle fibers; the difference in the configuration of the potentials is due to the position of the recording electrode.

FIRING PATTERN Qualitative and quantitative description of the sequence of discharge of potential waveforms recorded from muscle or nerve.

FIRING RATE Frequency of repetition of a potential. The relationship of the frequency to the occurrence of other potentials and the force of muscle contraction may be described. See *Discharge Frequency.*

FRACTIONATION OF MOTOR UNIT POTENTIALS Use of term discouraged. This term has been used to describe polyphasic, short-duration, low-amplitude motor unit potentials, a configuration thought to imply failure to activate all of the muscle fibers in a motor unit.

F REFLEX Use of term discouraged, as it is incorrect. No reflex is considered to be involved. See *F Wave.*

FREQUENCY Number of complete cycles of a repetitive waveform in 1 second. Measured in *Hertz* (Hz), a unit preferred to its equivalent, *Cycles Per Second* (C/sec).

FREQUENCY ANALYSIS Determination of the range of frequencies composing a potential waveform, with a measurement of the absolute or relative amplitude of each component frequency. It is similar to the mathematical technique of Fourier analysis.

F RESPONSE Synonymous with *F Wave.* See *F Wave.*

FULL INTERFERENCE PATTERN See *Interference Pattern.*

F WAVE A late compound action potential evoked intermittently from a muscle by a supramaximal electrical stimulus to the nerve.

Compared with the maximal amplitude M wave of the same muscle, the F wave has a reduced amplitude and variable configuration and a longer and more variable latency. It can be found in many muscles of the upper and lower extremities, and the latency is longer with more distal sites of stimulation. The *F* wave is due to antidromic activation of motor neurons. It was named by Magladery and McDougal in 1950. Contrast with *H Wave.*

G1, G2 Synonymous with Grid 1, Grid 2. See *Recording Electrodes.*

"GIANT" MOTOR UNIT ACTION POTENTIAL Use of term discouraged. It refers to a motor unit potential with a peak-to-peak amplitude and duration much greater than the range recorded in corresponding muscles in normal subjects of similar age. Quantitative measurements of amplitude and duration are preferable.

GROUND ELECTRODE An electrode connected to a large conducting body (such as the earth) used as a common return for an electrical circuit and as an arbitrary zero potential reference point.

GROUPED DISCHARGE Intermittent repetition of a group of *Action Potentials* with the same or nearly the same waveform and a relatively short interpotential interval within the group in comparison with the time interval between each group. It may occur spontaneously or with voluntary activity and may be regular or irregular in its firing pattern.

HABITUATION Decrease in amplitude and/or duration of a response with repeated stimuli. Response may be eliminated.

HERTZ (Abbr. Hz). Unit of frequency representing cycles per second.

HOFFMAN REFLEX See *H Wave*

H REFLEX Abbreviation for Hoffman reflex. See *H Wave.*

H RESPONSE Synonymous with *H Wave.*

H WAVE A late compound muscle action potential having a consistent latency evoked regularly, when present, from a muscle by an electrical stimulus to the nerve. It is regularly found only in a limited group of physiologic extensors, particularly the calf muscles. The reflex is most easily obtained with the cathode positioned proximal to the anode. Compared with the maximal amplitude *M Wave* of the same muscle, the H wave has a reduced amplitude, a longer latency, and a lower optimal stimulus intensity; its configuration is constant. The latency is longer with more distal sites of stimulation. A stimulus intensity sufficient to elicit a maximal-amplitude M wave reduces or abolishes the H wave. The H wave is thought to be due to a spinal reflex, the Hoffman reflex, with electrical stimulation of afferent fibers in the mixed nerve to the muscle and activation of motor neurons to the muscle through a monosynaptic connection in the spinal cord. The reflex and wave are named in honor of Hoffman's description (1918). Compare with *F Wave.*

HYPERPOLARIZATION See *Polarization.*

INCREASED INSERTIONAL ACTIVITY See *Insertional Activity.*

INCREMENTAL RESPONSE See synonym, *Incrementing Response.*

INCREMENTING RESPONSE A progressive increase in amplitude associated with an increase in the area of the negative phase of the *M Wave* of successive responses to a series of supramaximal stimuli. The rate of stimulation and the number of stimuli should be specified. Contrast with *Decrementing Response.*

INDIFFERENT ELECTRODE Synonymous with *Reference Electrode.* See *Recording Electrode.*

INHIBITORY POSTSYNAPTIC POTENTIAL (Abbr. *IPSP*). A local graded hyperpolarization of a neuron in response to activation at a synapse by a nerve terminal. Contrast with *Excitatory Postsynaptic Potential.*

INJURY POTENTIAL The potential difference between a normal region of the surface of a nerve or muscle and a region that has been injured; also called a demarcation potential. This potential was studied before intracellular recording was introduced. The injury potential approximates the potential across the membrane because the injured surface is almost at the potential of the inside of the cell. This term has been loosely used to describe *Insertional Activity* encountered in *Clinical Electromyography.*

INSERTIONAL ACTIVITY Electrical activity caused by insertion or movement of a needle electrode. The amount of the activity may be described qualitatively as *Normal, Reduced, Increased,* or *Prolonged.*

INTERDISCHARGE INTERVAL Time between consecutive discharges of the same potential. Measurements should be made between the corresponding points on each waveform.

INTERFERENCE Unwanted electrical activity arising outside the system being studied.

INTERFERENCE PATTERN Electrical activity recorded from a muscle with a needle electrode during maximal voluntary effort, in which identification of each of the contributing action potentials is not possible, because of the overlap or interference of one potential with another. When no individual potentials can be identified, this is known as a *Full Interference Pattern. A Reduced Interference Pattern* is one in which some of the individual potentials may be identified while other individual potentials cannot be identified because of overlapping. The term *Discrete Activity* is used to describe the electrical activity recorded when each of the motor unit potentials can be identified. It is important that the force of contraction associated with the interference pattern be specified.

INTERPOTENTIAL INTERVAL Time between two different potentials. Measurement should be made between the corresponding parts of each waveform.

INTRAMUSCULAR ELECTRODE An electrode usually used for recording and usually shaped like a needle to facilitate placement within a muscle belly.

INVOLUNTARY ACTIVITY Action potentials that are not under voluntary control. The condition under which they occur should be described, e.g., spontaneous, or, if elicited by a stimulus, the nature of the stimulus. Compare with *Spontaneous Activity.*

ISOELECTRIC DISCHARGE Recording obtained from a pair of equipotential electrodes.

ITERATIVE DISCHARGE See preferred term, *Repetitive Discharge.*

JITTER Synonymous with "single fiber electromyographic jitter." Jitter is the variability of the *Interpotential Interval* between two muscle fiber action potentials belonging to the same motor unit. It is usually expressed quantitatively as the mean value of the difference between the interpotential intervals of consecutive discharges (the mean consecutive difference, abbr. MCD). Under certain conditions, jitter is expressed as the mean value of the difference between the interpotential intervals arranged in the order of decreasing interpotential intervals (the mean sorted difference, abbr. MSD).

JOLLY TEST A technique, described in 1895 by Jolly, of application of a Faradic current to a motor nerve while recording the muscle contraction. This test has been refined and replaced by the technique of *Repetitive Stimulation* of motor nerves and the recording of successive M waves to detect a defect of neuromuscular transmission; use of the term is discouraged for modern testing techniques.

LATE COMPONENT OF A MOTOR UNIT POTENTIAL A potential separated from a *Motor Unit Potential* by a segment of baseline recording, but firing in a time-locked relationship to the motor unit potential.

LATE RESPONSE A general term used to describe an evoked potential having a longer latency than the *M Wave.* See *H Wave, F Wave.*

LATENCY Interval between the onset of a stimulus and the onset of a response unless otherwise specified. Latency always refers to the onset unless specified, as in *Peak Latency.*

LATENCY OF ACTIVATION The time required for an electrical stimulus to depolarize a nerve. In the past this had been estimated to be 0.1 msec.

LATENT PERIOD See synonym, *Latency.*

MALIGNANT FASCICULATION Use of term discouraged. See *Fasciculation Potential.*

MAXIMAL STIMULUS See *Stimulus.*

MAXIMAL NERVE CONDUCTION VELOCITY See *Conduction Velocity.*

MEMBRANE INSTABILITY Tendency of a cell membrane to depolarize spontaneously or after mechanical irritation or voluntary activation.

MICRONEUROGRAPHY The technique of recording peripheral nerve action potentials in man by means of intraneural microelectrodes.

MINIATURE END-PLATE POTENTIAL When recorded with microelectrodes, monophasic negative discharges with amplitudes less than 100 μV and duration of 4 msec or less, occurring irregularly and recorded in an area of muscle corresponding to the myoneural junction. They are thought to be due to small quantities (quanta) of acetylcholine released spontaneously. Compare with *End-Plate Activity.*

MIXED NERVE ACTION POTENTIAL See *Compound Nerve Action Potential.*

MONOPHASIC ACTION POTENTIAL An action potential with one phase.

MONOPHASIC END-PLATE ACTIVITY See *End-Plate Activity.*

MONOPOLAR NEEDLE ELECTRODE A solid wire, usually of stainless steel, coated, except at its tip, with an insulating material. Variations in voltage between the tip of the needle (active or exploring electrode) positioned in a muscle and a conductive plate on the skin surface or a bare needle in subcutaneous tissue (reference electrode) are measured. By convention, this recording condition is referred to as a monopolar needle electrode recording; it should be emphasized, however, that potential differences are always recorded between two electrodes.

MOTOR LATENCY Interval between the onset of a stimulus and the onset of the resultant *Compound Muscle Action Potential.* The term may be qualified as *Proximal Motor Latency* or *Distal Motor Latency,* depending on the relative position of the stimulus.

MOTOR NERVE ACTION POTENTIAL See *Compound Motor Nerve Action Potential.*

MOTOR NERVE CONDUCTION VELOCITY (Abbr. MNCV). See *Conduction Velocity.*

MOTOR POINT The point over a muscle where a contraction of a muscle may be elicited by a minimal-intensity, short-duration electrical stimulus.

MOTOR RESPONSE Either (1) the compound muscle action potential recorded over a muscle with stimulation of the nerve to the muscle or (2) the muscle twitch or contraction elicited by stimulation of the nerve to a muscle. As commonly used, the motor response refers only to the evoked potential, the *M Wave.*

MOTOR UNIT The anatomical unit of an anterior horn cell, its axon, the neuromuscular junctions, and all of the muscle fibers innervated by the axon.

MOTOR UNIT ACTION POTENTIAL (Abbr. MUAP). See synonym, *Motor Unit Potential.*

MOTOR UNIT POTENTIAL (Abbr. MUP). Action potential reflecting the electrical activity of that part of a single anatomical motor unit that is within the recording range of an electrode. The action potential is characterized by its consistent appearance with and relationship to the force of a voluntary contraction of a muscle. The following parameters should be specified, quantitatively if possible, after the recording electrode is placed so as to minimize the *Rise Time* (which by convention should be less than 0.5 msec), which generally also maximizes the amplitude:

I. Configuration
   A. *Amplitude,* peak-to-peak (μV or mV)
   B. *Duration,* total (msec)
   C. Number of *Phases* (*Monophasic, Biphasic, Triphasic, Tetraphasic, Polyphasic*)
   D. Direction of each *Phase* (negative, positive)
   E. Number of *Turns of Serrated Potential*
   F. Variation of shape with consecutive discharges
   G. Presence of *Late Components*

II. *Recruitment* characteristics
   A. Threshold of activation (first recruited, low threshold, high threshold)
   B. *Onset Frequency* (Hz)
   C. *Recruitment Frequency* (Hz) or *Recruitment Interval* (msec) of individual potentials

Descriptive terms implying diagnostic significance are not recommended, e.g., *Myopathic, Neuropathic, Regeneration, Nascent, Giant, BSAP,* and *BSAPP.*

MOTOR UNIT SUBUNIT Abandoned concept of muscle physiology. Fibers of a motor unit were considered to be arranged in groups of subunits containing an average of 10 fibers that fired synchronously. This is no longer accepted.

MOTOR UNIT TERRITORY (1) The area in which *Motor Unit Potentials* from a single motor unit may be recorded with a *Rise Time* of less than 0.5 msec. (2) The area in a muscle over which the muscle fibers of an individual motor unit are distributed anatomically.

MOVEMENT ARTIFACT See *Artifact.*

M RESPONSE See synonym, *M Wave.*

MUAP Abbreviation for motor unit action potential. See synonym, *Motor Unit Potential.*

MULTIELECTRODE See *Multilead Electrode.*

MULTILEAD ELECTRODE Three or more insulated wires inserted through a common metal cannula with their bared tips at an aperture in the cannula and flush with the outer circumference of the cannula. The arrangement of the bare tips relative to the axis of the cannula and the distance between each tip should be specified.

MULTIPLE DISCHARGE Four or more motor unit action potentials of the same form and nearly the same amplitude occurring consistently in the same relationship to one another. See *Double* and *Triple Discharge.*

MULTIPLET See *Multiple Discharge.*

MUP Abbreviation for *Motor Unit Potential.*

MUSCLE ACTION POTENTIAL Strictly defined, the term refers to the action potential recorded from a single muscle fiber. However, the term is commonly used to refer to a compound muscle action potential. See *Compound Muscle Action Potential.*

MUSCLE FIBER CONDUCTION VELOCITY The speed of propagation of a single muscle fiber action potential, usually expressed as meters per second. The muscle fiber conduction velocity is usually less than most nerve conduction velocities, varies with the rate of discharge of the muscle fiber, and requires special techniques for measurement.

MUSCLE UNIT An anatomical term referring to the group of muscle fibers innervated by a single motor neuron. See *Motor Unit.*

M WAVE *A Compound Action Potential* evoked from a muscle by a single electrical stimulus to its motor nerve. By convention, the M wave elicited by supramaximal stimulation is used for motor nerve conduction studies. The recording electrodes should be placed so that the initial deflection of the evoked potential is negative. The *Latency,* commonly called the *Motor Latency,* is the latency (milliseconds) to the onset of the first negative phase. The amplitude (millivolts) is the baseline-to-peak amplitude of the first negative phase, unless otherwise specified. The *Duration* (milliseconds) refers to the duration of the first negative phase, unless otherwise specified. Normally, the configuration of the M wave (usually biphasic) is quite stable with repeated stimuli at slow rates (1 to 5 Hz). See *Repetitive Stimulation.*

MYOKYMIA Involuntary, continuous quivering of muscle fibers which may be visible through the skin as a vermiform movement. It is associated with spontaneous, rhythmic discharge of *Motor Unit Potentials.* See *Myokymic Discharges, Fasciculation,* and *Fasciculation Potential.*

MYOKYMIC DISCHARGES Action potentials with the configuration of *Motor Unit Potentials* that occur spontaneously, recur regularly, and may be associated with clinical myokymia. Two distinct firing patterns are recognized. Commonly, the discharges are grouped with a short period (up to a few seconds) of firing at a uniform rate (2 to 20 Hz) followed by a short period (up to a few seconds) of silence, with repetition of the same sequence for a particular potential. Less commonly, the potential recurs continuously at a fairly uniform firing rate (1 to 5 Hz). Myokymic discharges are a subclass of *Grouped Discharges* and *Repetitive Discharges.*

MYOPATHIC MOTOR UNIT POTENTIAL Use of term discouraged. It is used to refer to low-amplitude, short-duration, polyphasic motor unit action potentials. The term incorrectly implies specific diagnostic significance of a motor unit potential configuration. See *Motor Unit Potential.*

MYOPATHIC RECRUITMENT Use of term discouraged. It is used to describe an increase in the number of and firing rate of motor unit potentials compared with normal for the strength of muscle contraction.

MYOTONIC DISCHARGE Repetitive discharge of 20 to 80 Hz of biphasic (positive-negative) spike potentials less than 5 msec in duration or monophasic positive waves of 5 to 20 msec recorded after needle insertion, or less commonly after voluntary muscle contraction or muscle percussion. The amplitude and frequency of the potentials must both wax and wane to be identified as myotonic discharges. This change produces a characteristic musical sound in the audio display of the electromyograph due to the corresponding change in pitch, which has been likened to the sound of a "dive bomber." Contrast with *Waning Discharge.*

MYOTONIC POTENTIAL See preferred term, *Myotonic Discharge.*

MYOTONIC RESPONSE Delayed relaxation of muscle after voluntary contraction or percussion and associated with a myotonic discharge. See *Myotonic Discharge.*

NASCENT MOTOR UNIT POTENTIAL From the Latin *nascens,* to be born. Use of term is discouraged as it incorrectly implies diagnostic significance of a motor unit potential configuration. Term has been used to refer to very low-amplitude, long-duration, highly polyphasic motor unit potentials observed during early stages of reinnervation of muscle. See *Motor Unit Potential.*

NASCENT UNIT Use of term discouraged. See *Nascent Motor Unit Potential.*

NEEDLE ELECTRODE An electrode for recording or stimulating, shaped like a needle. See specific electrodes: *Bipolar Needle Electrode, Concentric Needle Electrode, Monopolar Needle Electrode, Multilead Electrode.*

NERVE ACTION POTENTIAL Strictly defined, refers to an action potential recorded from a single nerve fiber. The term is commonly used to refer to the compound nerve action potential. See *Compound Nerve Action Potential.*

NERVE CONDUCTION STUDIES Refers to all aspects of electrodiagnostic studies of peripheral nerves. However, the term is generally used to refer to the recording and measurement of *Compound Nerve* and *Compound Muscle Action Potentials* elicited in response to a single supramaximal electrical *Stimulus* under standardized conditions that permit establishment of normal ranges of amplitude, duration, and latency of *Evoked Potentials* and the calculation of the *Maximum Conduction Velocity* of individual nerves. See *Compound Nerve Action Potential, Compound Muscle Action Potential, Conduction Velocity,* and *Repetitive Stimulation.*

NERVE CONDUCTION VELOCITY (Abbr. NCV). Loosely used to refer to the maximum nerve conduction velocity. See *Conduction Velocity.*

NERVE POTENTIAL Equivalent to *Nerve Action Potential.* Also commonly, but inaccurately, used to refer to the biphasic form of *End-Plate Activity.* The latter use is incorrect because muscle fibers, not nerve fibers, are the source of these potentials.

NERVE TRUNK ACTION POTENTIAL See preferred term, *Compound Nerve Action Potential.*

NEUROMYOTONIA Clinical syndrome of continuous muscle fiber activity manifested as continuous muscle rippling and stiffness. It may be associated with a variety of electrical discharges.

NEUROMYOTONIC DISCHARGES Bursts of *Motor Unit Potentials* firing at more than 150 Hz for ½ to 2 sec. The amplitude of the response typically wanes. Discharges may occur spontaneously or be initiated by needle movement.

NEUROPATHIC MOTOR UNIT POTENTIAL Use of term discouraged. It is used to refer to abnormally high-amplitude, long-duration, polyphasic *Motor Unit Potentials.* The term incorrectly implies a specific diagnostic significance of a motor unit potential configuration. See *Motor Unit Potential.*

NEUROPATHIC RECRUITMENT Use of term discouraged. It has been used to describe a recruitment pattern with a decreased number of *Motor Unit Potentials* firing at a rapid rate. See preferred terms, *Discrete Activity, Reduced Interference Pattern.*

NOISE Strictly defined, an *Artifact* consisting of low-amplitude, random potentials produced by an amplifier and unrelated to the input signal. It is most apparent when high gains are used. It is loosely used to refer to end-plate noise. Compare with *End-Plate Activity.*

ONSET FREQUENCY The lowest stable frequency of firing for a single *Motor Unit Potential* that can be voluntarily maintained by a subject.

ONSET LATENCY Tautology. See *Latency.*

ORDER OF ACTIVATION The sequence of appearance of different *Motor Unit Potentials* with increasing strength of voluntary contraction. See *Recruitment.*

ORTHODROMIC Said of *Action Potentials* or stimuli eliciting action potentials propagated in the same direction as physiological conduction, e.g., motor nerve conduction away from the spinal cord and sensory nerve conduction toward the spinal cord. Contrast with *Antidromic.*

PAIRED DISCHARGE Two action potentials of the same form and nearly the same amplitude occurring consistently in the same relationship to each other at intervals of 20 to 80 msec. Contrast with *Double Discharge.*

PAIRED RESPONSE Loosely used to refer to either the preferred term *Paired Discharge* or the preferred term *Late Component.*

PAIRED STIMULI Two temporally linked stimuli. The time interval between the two stimuli and the intensity of each stimulus should be specified. The first is called the *Conditioning Stimulus* and the second the *Test Stimulus.*

PARASITE POTENTIAL See preferred term, *Late Component of a Motor Unit Potential.*

PEAK LATENCY Interval between the onset of a stimulus and a specified peak of the evoked potential (usually the negative peak).

PHASE That portion of a *Wave* between the departure from and the return to the *Baseline.*

POLARIZATION As used in neurophysiology, the presence of an electrical *Potential* difference across an excitable cell membrane. The potential across the membrane of a cell when it is not excited by input or spontaneously active is termed the *Resting Potential;* it is at a steady state with regard to the electrical potential difference across the membrane. *Depolarization* describes a decrease in polarization to any degree, relative to the normal resting potential. *Hyperpolarization* describes an increase in polarization relative to the resting potential. *Repolarization* describes an increase in polarization from the depolarized state toward, but not above, the normal or resting potential.

POLYPHASIC ACTION POTENTIAL An *Action Potential* having five or more phases. See *Phase.* Contrast with *Serrated Action Potential.*

POSITIVE SHARP WAVE Strictly defined, one form of electrical activity associated with fibrillating muscle fibers. It is recorded as a biphasic, positive-negative *Action Potential* initiated by needle movement and recurring in a uniform, regular pattern at a rate of 2 to 50 Hz, which may decrease just before cessation of discharge. The amplitude and duration vary considerably but the initial positive deflection is usually less than 5 msec in duration and up to 1 mV in amplitude. The negative phase is of low amplitude, with a duration of 10-100 msec. A sequence of positive sharp waves is commonly referred to as a *Train of Positive Sharp Waves.* Positive sharp waves are recorded from the damaged area of fibrillating muscle fibers. Loosely defined, positive sharp waves refer to any action potential recorded with the waveform of a positive wave, without reference to the firing pattern or method of generation.

POSITIVE WAVE Strictly defined, the positive phase of a waveform. Loosely defined, the term refers to a positive sharp wave. See *Positive Sharp Wave.*

POSTACTIVATION DEPRESSION The reduction in the amplitude of an *Evoked Potential* in response to a single *Stimulus* which occurs after *Repetitive Stimulation* or after voluntary contraction.

POSTACTIVATION EXHAUSTION The reduction of the amplitude associated with a decrease in the area of the negative phase of the initial *M Wave* and/or the exaggeration of the *Decrementing Response* seen 2 to 4 min after either a brief (10 to 30 sec), strong voluntary contraction or a period of nerve stimulation causing tetanic muscle contraction. Compare with *Postactivation Facilitation.*

POSTACTIVATION FACILITATION The increase in amplitude associated with an increase in the area of the negative phase of the initial *M Wave* and/or the diminution of the *Decrementing Response* seen a few seconds after either a brief (10 to 30 sec), strong voluntary contraction or a period of nerve stimulation causing tetanic muscle contraction. Compare with *Postactivation Exhaustion.*

POSTACTIVATION POTENTIATION Synonymous with preferred term, *Postactivation Facilitation.*

POSTTETANIC POTENTIATION Enhancement of excitability following a long period of high-frequency stimulation. This phenomenon is known mainly in the mammalian spinal cord, where it lasts minutes or even hours. Use of the term is not recommended to describe the phenomenon of *Postactivation Facilitation.*

POTENTIAL Strictly, *Voltage;* loosely, synonymous with *Action Potential.* See *Polarization.*

PROLONGED INSERTIONAL ACTIVITY See *Insertional Activity.*

PROPAGATION VELOCITY OF A MUSCLE FIBER The speed of transmission of a muscle fiber action potential.

PROXIMAL LATENCY See *Motor Latency* and *Sensory Latency.*

PSEUDOFACILITATION (OF NEUROMUSCULAR TRANSMISSION) Use of term discouraged. It refers to an increase in amplitude with a corresponding reduction in duration of the negative phase of the *M Wave,* resulting in no change in the area of the negative phase of the M wave. This probably reflects a reduction in the temporal dispersion of a constant number of summated muscle fiber action potentials, and must be differentiated from *Postactivation Facilitation.* See *Postactivation Facilitation.*

PSEUDOMYOTONIC DISCHARGE Use of term discouraged. It has been used to refer to different phenomena, including (1) *Myotonic Discharges* occurring in the presence of a neurogenic disease, (2) *Complex Repetitive Discharges,* and (3) *Repetitive Discharges* that wax or wane in either frequency or amplitude but not in both. See *Waning Discharge.*

PSEUDOPOLYPHASIC ACTION POTENTIAL Use of term discouraged. See preferred term, *Serrated Action Potential.*

R1, R2 WAVES See *Blink Responses.*

RECORDING ELECTRODE Device used to monitor electrical current or potential. All electrical recordings require two *Electrodes.* The electrode close to the source of the activity to be recorded is called the *Active* or *Exploring Electrode,* and the other electrode is called the *Reference Electrode.* Active electrode is synonymous with the older terminology G1 or Grid 1, and the reference electrode with G2 or Grid 2. By current convention, a potential difference that is negative at the active electrode relative to the reference electrode causes an upward deflection on the oscilloscope screen. The term "monopolar recording" is not recommended, because all recording requires two electrodes; however, it is commonly used to describe the use of an intramuscular needle exploring electrode in combination with a surface disc or subcutaneous needle reference electrode.

RECRUITMENT The orderly activation of the same and new motor units with increasing strength of voluntary muscle contraction. See *Motor Unit Potential.*

RECRUITMENT FREQUENCY Firing rate of a *Motor Unit Potential* when an additional motor unit potential first appears during gradually increasing strength of voluntary muscle contraction.

RECRUITMENT INTERVAL The *Interdischarge Interval* between two consecutive discharges of a *Motor Unit Potential* when an additional motor unit potential first appears during gradually increasing strength of voluntary muscle contraction. The reciprocal of the recruitment interval is the *Recruitment Frequency.*

RECRUITMENT PATTERN A qualitative and/or quantitative description of the sequence of appearance of *Motor Unit Potentials* with increasing strength of voluntary muscle contraction. The *Recruitment Frequency* and *Recruitment Interval* are two quantitative measures commonly used. See *Interference Pattern* for qualitative terms commonly used.

REDUCED INSERTIONAL ACTIVITY See *Insertional Activity.*

REDUCED INTEREFERENCE PATTERN See *Interference Pattern.*

REFERENCE ELECTRODE—See *Recording Electrode.*

REFLEX A stereotyped *Motor Response* elicited by a *Stimulus.*

REFRACTORY PERIOD Time after an *Action Potential* during which the response to an additional stimulus is altered. The *Absolute Refractory Period* is that segment of the refractory period during which no stimulus, however strong, evokes an additional action potential. The *Relative Refractory Period* is that segment of the refractory period during which a stimulus must be greater than a normal threshold stimulus to evoke a second action potential.

RELATIVE REFRACTORY PERIOD See *Refractory Period.*

REPETITIVE DISCHARGES General term for the recurrence of an *Action Potential* with the same or nearly the same form. The term may refer to recurring potentials recorded in muscle at rest, during voluntary contraction, or in response to single nerve stimulus. The discharge may be named for the number of times a potential recurs in a group (e.g., *Double Discharge, Triple Discharge, Multiple Discharge, Coupled Discharge*) or other characteristics (e.g., *Complex Repetitive Discharge, Myokymic Discharge*).

REPETITIVE STIMULATION The technique of utilizing repeated supramaximal stimulation of a nerve while quantitatively recording *M Waves* from muscles innervated by the nerve. It should be described in terms of the frequency of stimuli and number of stimuli (or duration of the total group). For descriptions of specific patterns of responses, see the terms *Incrementing Response, Decrementing Response, Postactivation Facilitation,* and *Postactivation Exhaustion.*

REPOLARIZATION See *Polarization.*

RESIDUAL LATENCY Refers to the calculated time difference between the measured distal latency of a motor nerve and the expected distal latency, calculated by dividing the distance between the stimulus cathode and the active recording electrode by the maximum conduction velocity measured in a more proximal segment of a nerve.

RESPONSE Used to describe an activity elicited by a *Stimulus.*

RESTING MEMBRANE POTENTIAL Voltage across the membrane of an excitable cell at rest. See *Polarization.*

RHEOBASE The intensity of an electrical current of infinitely long duration necessary to produce a minimal visible twitch of a muscle when the cathode is applied to the motor point of the muscle. In practice a duration of at least 300 msec is used to determine the rheobase.

RISE TIME By convention, the shortest interval from the nadir of a positive phase to the peak of a negative phase of a *Wave.*

SATELLITE POTENTIAL Synonymous with preferred term, *Late Component.*

SEA SHELL NOISE (SEE SHELL ROAR) Use of term discouraged. See *End-Plate Activity, Monophasic.*

SENSORY DELAY See preferred terms, *Sensory Latency* and *Sensory Peak Latency.*

SENSORY LATENCY Interval between the onset of a stimulus and the onset of the *Compound Sensory Nerve Action Potential.* This term has been loosely used to refer to the *Sensory Peak Latency.* The term may be qualified as *Proximal Sensory Latency* or *Distal Sensory Latency,* depending on the relative position of the stimulus.

SENSORY NERVE ACTION POTENTIAL See *Compound Sensory Nerve Action Potential.*

SENSORY NERVE CONDUCTION VELOCITY See *Conduction Velocity.*

SENSORY PEAK LATENCY Interval between the onset of a *Stimulus* and the peak of the negative phase of the *Compound Sensory Nerve Action Potential.* Note that the term "*Latency*" refers to the interval between the onset of a stimulus and the onset of a response.

SENSORY POTENTIAL Used to refer to the compound sensory nerve action potential. See *Compound Sensory Nerve Action Potential.*

SENSORY RESPONSE Used to refer to a sensory evoked potential, e.g., *Compound Sensory Nerve Action Potential.*

SERRATED ACTION POTENTIAL An action potential waveform with several changes in direction (turns) which do not cross the baseline. This term is preferred to the terms *Complex Action Potential* and *Pseudopolyphasic Action Potential.* See *Turns.*

SHOCK ARTIFACT See *Artifact.*

SILENT PERIOD Time during which there is no electrical activity in muscle following rapid unloading of a muscle.

SINGLE-FIBER ELECTROMYOGRAPHY (Abbr. SFEMG). General term referring to the technique and conditions that permit recording of a single muscle fiber *Action Potential.* See *Single-Fiber Needle Electrode.*

SINGLE-FIBER NEEDLE ELECTRODE A needle *Electrode* with a small recording surface (usually 25 μm in diameter) permitting the recording of single muscle fiber action potentials. See *Single-Fiber Electromyography.*

SOMATOSENSORY EVOKED POTENTIAL (Abbr. SSEP). Electrical *Waves* recorded from the head or trunk in response to electrical or physiological stimulation of peripheral sensory fibers. Recordings over the spine may be referred to as *Spinal Evoked Potentials.*

SPIKE Transient *Wave* with a pointed peak and a short duration (a few milliseconds or less). See *End-Plate Spike* and *Fibrillation Potentials.*

SPINAL EVOKED POTENTIAL Electrical *Wave* recorded over the spine in response to electrical stimulation of peripheral sensory fibers. See *Somatosensory Evoked Potential.*

SPONTANEOUS ACTIVITY Action potentials recorded from muscle or nerve at rest after insertional activity has subsided and when there is no voluntary contraction or external stimulus. Compare with *Involuntary Activity.*

STAIRCASE PHENOMENON The progressive increase in the force of a muscle contraction observed with repeated nerve stimulation at low rates.

STIGMATIC ELECTRODE Synonymous with active or exploring electrode. See *Recording Electrodes.*

STIMULATING ELECTRODE Device used to apply electrical current. All electrical stimulation requires two electrodes; the negative terminal is termed the *Cathode* and the positive terminal, the *Anode.* By convention, the stimulating electrodes are called "*Bipolar*" if they are roughly equal in size and separated by less than 5 cm. The stimulating electrodes are called "*Monopolar*" if the cathode is smaller in size than the anode and is separated from the anode by more than 5 cm. Electrical stimulation for *Nerve Conduction Studies* generally requires application of the cathode to produce depolarization of the nerve trunk fibers. If the anode is inadvertently placed between the cathode and the recording electrodes, a focal block of nerve conduction (*Anodal Block*) may occur and cause a technically unsatisfactory study.

STIMULUS Any external agent, state, or change that is capable of influencing the activity of a cell, tissue, or organism. In clinical *Nerve Conduction Studies,* an electrical stimulus is generally applied to a nerve or a muscle. The electrical stimulus may be described in absolute terms or with respect to the evoked potential of the nerve or muscle. In absolute terms, the electrical stimulus has a strength or intensity measured in voltage (volts) or current (milliamperes) and a duration (milliseconds). With respect to the evoked potential, the stimulus may be graded as subthreshold, threshold, submaximal, maximal, or supramaximal. A *Threshold Stimulus* is that electrical stimulus just sufficient to produce a detectable response. Stimuli less than the threshold stimulus are termed *Subthreshold.* The *Maximal Stimulus* is the stimulus intensity after which a further increase in the stimulus intensity causes no increase in the amplitude of the evoked potential. Stimuli of intensity below this and above threshold are *Submaximal.* Stimuli of intensity greater than the maximal stimulus are termed *Supramaximal.* Ordinarily, supramaximal stimuli are used for nerve conduction studies. By convention, an electrical stimulus of approximately 20% greater voltage than required for the maximal stimulus may be used for supramaximal stimulation. The frequency, number, and duration of a series of stimuli should be specified.

STIMULUS ARTIFACT See *Artifact.*

STRENGTH-DURATION CURVE Graphic presentation of the relationship between the intensity (Y axis) and various durations (X axis) of the threshold electrical stimulus for a muscle with the stimulating cathode positioned over the motor point.

SUBMAXIMAL STIMULUS See *Stimulus.*

SUBTHRESHOLD STIMULUS See *Stimulus.*

SUPRAMAXIMAL STIMULUS See *Stimulus.*

SURFACE ELECTRODE Conducting device for stimulating or recording placed on a skin surface. The material (Metal, fabric), configuration (disc, ring), size, and separation should be specified. See *Electrode* (*Ground, Recording, Stimulating*).

S-X INTERVAL The total duration of the *Silent Period* produced by electrical stimulation of the mixed nerve to a voluntarily contracting muscle, measured from the stimulus artifact to resumption of uninterrupted voluntary activity.

TEMPORAL DISPERSION A waveform of longer duration than normal. Commonly used to refer to an increase in the duration of an evoked potential with more proximal sites of stimulation of a greater degree than that normally seen.

TERMINAL LATENCY Synonymous with preferred term, *Distal Latency.* See *Motor Latency* and *Sensory Latency.*

TEST STIMULUS The stimulus producing the event being measured. Contrast with *Conditioning Stimulus.*

TETANIC CONTRACTION State of a muscle in sustained contraction resulting from stimulation at a frequency high enough for individual twitches to summate to a smooth tension and with associated electrical activity of muscle action potentials. It may be attained in normal muscle voluntarily or in response to repetitive nerve stimulation. Contrast with *Cramp Discharge.*

TETANUS Loosely used to refer to *Tetanic Contraction.* The term is also used to refer to the acute infectious disease. See *Tetanic Contraction* and *Tetany.*

TETANY A clinical syndrome manifested by muscle twitching, cramps, and sustained muscle contraction (*Tetanus*). These clinical signs are manifestations of peripheral and central nervous system nerve irritability from several causes. In these conditions, *Repetitive Discharges* (double discharge, triple discharge, multiple discharge) occur frequently with voluntary activation of motor unit potentials or may appear as spontaneous activity with systemic alkalosis or local ischemia.

TETRAPHASIC ACTION POTENTIAL *Action Potential* with four phases.

THRESHOLD The level at which a clear and abrupt transition occurs from one state to another. The term is generally used to refer to the voltage level at which an *Action Potential* is initiated in a single axon or a group of axons. It is also operationally defined as the intensity that produced a response in about 50% of equivalent trials.

THRESHOLD STIMULUS See *Stimulus.*

TIME CONSTANT OF ACCOMMODATION (lambda, λ). The time constant of the rate at which, after accommodation, the threshold of an excitable tissue reverts to its initial level. It is the reciprocal of the slope of the *Accommodation Curve.*

TRAIN OF POSITIVE SHARP WAVES See *Positive Sharp Waves.*

TRAIN OF STIMULI A group of stimuli. The duration of the group and the frequency of the individual components should be specified.

TRIPHASIC ACTION POTENTIAL *Action Potential* with three phases.

TRIPLE DISCHARGE Three action potentials of the same form and nearly the same amplitude, occurring consistently in the same relationship to one another. The interval between the second and the third action potential often exceeds that between the first two, and both are usually in the range of 2-20 msec.

TRIPLET See *Triple Discharge.*

TURNS Changes in direction of a waveform which do not necessarily pass through the baseline. The minimal excursion required to constitute a turn should be specified.

UNIPOLAR NEEDLE ELECTRODE See synonym, *Monopolar Needle Electrode.*

VISUAL EVOKED POTENTIAL Electrical waveforms of biological origin recorded over the cerebrum and elicited by light stimuli.

VISUAL EVOKED RESPONSE (Abbr. VER). See *Visual Evoked Potential.*

VOLTAGE Potential difference between two points.

VOLUME CONDUCTION Spread of current from a potential source through a conducting medium, such as the body tissues.

VOLUNTARY ACTIVITY In electromyography, the electrical activity recorded from a muscle with consciously controlled muscle contraction. The effort made to contract the muscle, e.g., minimal, moderate, or maximal, and the strength of contraction in absolute terms or relative to a maximal voluntary contraction of a normal corresponding muscle should be specified.

WANING DISCHARGE General term referring to a repetitive discharge that decreases in frequency or in amplitude. Compare with *Myotonic Discharge.*

WAVE An undulating line constituting a graphic representation of a change, e.g., a changing electrical potential difference.

WAVEFORM The shape of a *Wave.* The term is often used synonymously with wave.

WEDENSKY-LIKE NEUROMUSCULAR FAILURE Use of term discouraged. The term has been used to describe a decrease in the strength of the sustained muscle contraction during repeated nerve stimulation at frequencies within the physiological range (less than 50 Hz). See preferred term, *Decrementing Response.*

WEDENSKY PHENOMENON A decrease in strength of a sustained muscle contraction during sustained nerve stimulation at frequencies above the physiological range, e.g., greater than 50 Hz. This phenomenon is seen in normal muscle.

Bibliography

Baer RD, Johnson EW: Motor nerve conduction velocities in normal children. *Arch Phys Med Rehabil* 46:698–704, 1965.

Behse F, Buchthal F: Normal sensory conduction in the nerves of the leg in man. *J. Neurol Neurosurg Psychiatry* 34:404–414, 1971.

Bhala RP, Goodgold J: Motor conduction in the deep palmar branch of the ulnar nerve. *Arch Phys Med Rehabil* 49:460–466, 1968.

Braddom RL, Johnson EW: H reflex: Review and classification with suggested clinical uses. *Arch Phys Med Rehabil* 55:412–417, 1974.

Braddom RL, Johnson EW: Standardization of H reflex and diagnostic use in S1 radiculopathy. *Arch Phys Med Rehabil* 55:161–166, 1974.

Buchthal F: Electrophysiological findings in entrapment of the median nerve of wrist and elbow. *J. Neurol Neurosurg Psychiatry* 37:340–360, 1974.

Buchthal F, Rosenfalck A: Evoked action potentials and conduction velocity in human sensory nerve. *Brain Res* 3:1–119, 1966.

Buchthal F, Rosenfalck A, Tojaborg W: Electrophysiological findings in entrapment of the median nerve at wrist and elbow. *J. Neurol Neurosurg Psychiatry* 37:340–360, 1974.

Butler ET, Johnson EW, Kaye ZA: Normal conduction velocity in the lateral femoral cutaneous nerve. *Arch Phys Med Rehabil* 55:31–32, 1974.

Cerra D, Johnson EW: Motor conduction velocity in premature infants. *Arch Phys Med Rehabil* 43:160–164, 1962.

Checkles NS, Bailey JA, Johnson EW: Tape and caliper surface measurements in determination of peroneal nerve conduction velocity. *Arch Phys Med Rehabil* 50:214–218, 1969.

Checkles NS, Russakov AD, Piero DL: Ulnar nerve conduction velocity: Effect of elbow position on measurement. *Arch Phys Med Rehabil* 52:362–365, 1971.

Cherington M: Accessory nerve. Conduction studies. *Arch Neurol* 18:708–709, 1968.

Clay SA, Ramseyer JC: The orbicularis oculi reflex in infancy and childhood. *Neurology (Minneap)* 26:521–524, 1976.

Davis JN: Phrenic nerve conduction in man. *J. Neurol Neurosurg Psychiatry* 30:420–426, 1967.

Desmedt JE: The neuromuscular disorder in myasthenia gravis. In *New Developments in Electromyography and Clinical Neurophysiology, Vol. 1,* edited by JE Desmedt, pp. 241–342, S Karger AG, Basel, 1973.

Desmedt JE, Borenstein S: Diagnosis of myasthenia gravis by nerve stimulation. *Ann NY Acad Sci* 274:174–188, 1976.

Devi S, Lovelace RE, Duarte N: Proximal peroneal nerve conduction velocity: Recording from anterior tibial and peroneus brevis muscles. *Ann Neurol* 2:116–119, 1977.

DiBenedetto M: Sensory nerve conduction in lower extremities. *Arch Phys Med Rehabil* 51:253–258 passim, 1970.

Dick HC, Bradley WE, Scott FB, Timm GW: Pudendal sexual reflexes. Electrophysiologic investigations. *Urology* 3:376–379, 1974.

Feibel A, Foca FJ: Sensory conduction of radial nerve. *Arch Phys Med Rehabil* 55:314–316, 1974.

Fu R, DeLisa JA, Kraft GH: Motor nerve latencies through the tarsal tunnel in normal adult subjects: Standard determinations corrected for temperature and distance. *Arch Phys Med Rehabil* 61:243–248, 1980.

Gamstorp I: Normal conduction velocity of ulnar, median and peroneal nerves in infancy, childhood, and adolescence. *Acta Paediatr Scand (Suppl)* 146:68–76, 1963.

Gamstorp I, Shelburne SA: Peripheral sensory conduction in ulnar and median nerves of normal infants, children and adolescents. *Acta Paediatr Scand* 54:309–313, 1965.

Gassel MM: A study of femoral nerve conduction time. *Arch Neurol* 9:607–614, 1963.

Jebsen RH: Motor conduction velocity of distal radial nerve. *Arch Phys Med Rehabil* 47:12–16, 1966.

Jebsen RH: Motor conduction velocity in proximal and distal segments of the radial nerve. *Arch Phys Med Rehabil* 47:597–602, 1966.

Jimenez J, Easton JK, Redford JB: Conduction studies of the anterior and posterior tibial nerves. *Arch Phys Med Rehabil* 51:164–169, 1970.

Johnson EW, Melvin JL: Sensory conduction studies of median and ulnar nerves. *Arch Phys Med Rehabil* 48:25–30, 1967.

Johnson EW, Ortiz PR: Electrodiagnosis of tarsal tunnel syndrome. *Arch Phys Med Rehabil* 47:776–780, 1966.

Johnson EW, Wood PK, Powers JJ: Femoral nerve conduction studies. *Arch Phys Med Rehabil* 49:528–532, 1968.

Kaplan PE: Electrodiagnostic confirmation of long thoracic nerve palsy. *J. Neurol Neurosurg Psychiatry* 43:50–52, 1980.

Kimura J: Collision technique: Physiologic block of nerve impulses in studies of motor nerve conduction velocity. *Neurology (Minneap)* 26:680–682, 1976.

Kimura J: F-wave velocity in the central segment of the median and ulnar nerves. A study in normal subjects and in patients with Charcot-Marie-Tooth disease. *Neurology (Minneap)* 24:539–546, 1974.

Kimura J, Bokensteiner J, Yamada T: Electrically elicited blink reflex in normal neonates. *Arch Neurol* 34:246–249, 1977.

Kimura J, Bosch P, Lindsay GM: F-wave conduction velocity in the central segment of the peroneal and tibial nerves. *Arch Phys Med Rehabil* 56:492–497, 1975.

Kimura J, Giron LT, Young SM: Electrophysiological study of Bell palsy. *Arch Otolaryngol* 102:140–143, 1976.

Kraft GH: Axillary, musculocutaneous and suprascapular nerve latency studies. *Arch Phys Med Rehabil* 53:383–387, 1972.

Lambert EH: The accessory deep peroneal nerve. A common variation in innervation of extensor digitorum brevis. *Neurology (Minneap)* 19:1169–1176, 1969.

Lambert EH, Rooke ED: Myasthenic state and lung cancer. In: Brain WR, Norris FH (eds): *Remote Effects of Cancer on the Nervous System.* New York, Grune & Stratton, 1965, pp 67–80.

Lovelace RE, Myers SJ, Zablow L: Sensory conduction in peroneal and posterior tibial nerves using averaging techniques. *J. Neurol Neurosurg Psychiatry* 36:942–950, 1973.

Mackenzie K, DeLisa JA: Determining the distal sensory latency of the superficial radial nerve in normal adult subjects. *Arch Phys Med Rehabil* 62:31–34, 1981.

MacLean IC: Nerve root stimulation to evaluate conduction across the brachial and lumbosacral plexus. Recent advances in clinical electromyography. *AAEE Third Anual Continuing Education Course* 51–55, Sept 1980.

Melvin JL, Harris DH, Johnson EW: Sensory and motor conduction velocities in the ulnar and median nerves. *Arch Phys Med Rehabil* 47:511–519, 1966.

Melvin JL, Schuchmann JA, Lanese RR: Diagnostic specificity of motor and sensory nerve conduction variables in the carpal tunnel syndrome. *Arch Phys Med Rehabil* 54:69–74, 1973.

Oh SJ: Botulism: Electrophysiological studies. *Ann Neurol* 1:481–485, 1977.

Oh SJ, Sarala PK, Kuba T, Elmore RS: Tarsal tunnel syndrome: Electrophysiological study. *Ann Neurol* 5:327–330, 1979.

Panayiotopoulos CP, Scarpalezos S, Nastas PE: F-wave studies in the deep peroneal nerve. Part 1. Control subjects. *J Neurol Sci* 31:319–329, 1977.

Panayiotopoulos CP, Scarpalezos S, Nastas PE: Sensory (Ia) and F-wave conduction velocity in the proximal segment of the tibial nerve. *Muscle Nerve* 1:181–189, 1978.

Pribyl R, You SB, Jantra P: Sensory nerve conduction velocity of the medial antebrachial cutaneous nerve. *Electromyogr Clin Neurophysiol* 19:41–46, 1979.

Sarala PK, Nishihara T, Oh SJ: Meralgia paresthetica: Electrophysiologic study. *Arch Phys Med Rehabil* 60:30–31, 1979.

Schuchmann JA: Sural nerve conduction: A standardized technique. *Arch Phys Med Rehabil* 58:166–168, 1977.

Siroky MB, Sax DS, Krane RJ: Sacral signal tracing: The electrophysiology of the bulbocavernosus reflex. *J Urol* 122:661–664, 1979.

Spindler HA, Felsenthal G: Sensory conduction in the musculocutaneous nerve. *Arch Phys Med Rehabil* 59:20–23, 1978.

Taylor N, Jebsen RH, Tenckhoff HA: Facial nerve conduction latency in chronic renal insufficiency. *Arch Phys Med Rehabil* 51:259–263, 1970.

Tojaborg W: Motor and sensory conduction in the musculocutaneous nerve. *J. Neurol Neurosurg Psychiatry* 39:890–899, 1976.

Trojaborg W, Sindrup EG: Motor and sensory conduction in different segments of the radial nerve in normal subjects. *J Neurol Neurosurg Psychiatry* 32:354–359, 1969.

Truong XT, Russo FI, Vagi I, Rippel DV: Conduction velocity in the proximal sural nerve. *Arch Phys Med Rehabil* 60:304–308, 1979.

Wagner AL, Buchthal F: Motor and sensory conduction in infancy and childhood: Reappraisal. *Dev Med Child Neurol* 14:189–216, 1972.

Wainapel SF, Kim DJ, Ebel A: Conduction studies of the saphenous nerve in healthy subjects. *Arch Phys Med Rehabil* 59:316–319, 1978.

Waylonis GW, Johnson EW: Facial nerve conduction velocity. *Arch Phys Med Rehabil* 45:539–547, 1964.

Wiederholt WC: Stimulus intensity and site of excitation in human median nerve sensory fibres. *J Neurol Neurosurg Psychiatry* 33:438–441, 1970.

Wilbourn AJ, Lambert EH: The forearm median-to-ulnar nerve communication: Electrodiagnostic aspects. *Neurology (Minneap)* 26:368, 1976.

Yap C-B, Hirota T: Sciatic nerve motor conduction velocity study. *J Neurol Neurosurg Psychiatry* 30:233–239, 1967.

Subject Index